DIGITAL RADIOGRAPHY
AND PACS

DIGITAL RADIOGRAPHY AND PACS

REVISED

Christi E. Carter, MSRS, RT(R)
Professor and Director
Radiologic Sciences Program
Brookhaven College
Farmers Branch, Texas

Beth L. Vealé, M.Ed., RT(R)(QM)
Associate Professor of Radiologic Sciences
Midwestern State University
Wichita Falls, Texas

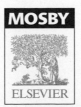

MOSBY

ELSEVIER

11830 Westline Industrial Drive
St. Louis, Missouri 63146

DIGITAL RADIOGRAPHY AND PACS ISBN: 978–0–323–07221–2

Notice

Knowledge and best practice in this field are constantly changing. As new research and experience broaden our knowledge, changes in practice, treatment and drug therapy may become necessary or appropriate. Readers are advised to check the most current information provided (i) on procedures featured or (ii) by the manufacturer of each product to be administered, to verify the recommended dose or formula, the method and duration of administration, and contraindications. It is the responsibility of the practitioner, relying on their own experience and knowledge of the patient, to make diagnoses, to determine dosages and the best treatment for each individual patient, and to take all appropriate safety precautions. To the fullest extent of the law, neither the Publisher nor the Editors/Authors assume any liability for any injury and/or damage to persons or property arising out of or related to any use of the material contained in this book.

The Publisher

Library of Congress Cataloging-in-Publication Data

Carter, Christi E.
  Digital radiography and PACS / Christi E. Carter, Beth L. Vealé. -- 1st ed., rev.
    p. ; cm.
  Includes index.
  ISBN 978-0-323-07221-2 (pbk. : alk. paper)   1. Radiography, Medical--Digital techniques.   2. Picture archiving and communication systems in medicine. I. Vealé, Beth L. II. Title.
   [DNLM: 1. Image Processing, Computer-Assisted--methods. 2. Radiographic Image Interpretation, Computer-Assisted--instrumentation. 3. Radiographic Image Interpretation, Computer-Assisted--methods. WN 26.5 C323d 2010]
  RC78.7.D35C37 2010
  616.07'572–dc22   2009019833

Publisher: Jeanne Olson
Senior Developmental Editor: Linda Woodard
Editorial Assistant: Luke Held
Publishing Services Manager: Pat Joiner-Myers
Senior Project Manager: David Stein
Design Direction: Kim Denando

Printed in Canada

Last digit is the print number: 9 8 7 6 5 4 3 2 1

Reviewers

To
Our families
and
Colleagues too numerous to name

Preface

Digital imaging is not new; in fact, it has been in constant development since the 1960's. Despite that, its arrival on the diagnostic imaging scene was a bit of a surprise to most imaging technologists. Computed tomography, magnetic resonance imaging, and ultrasound have utilized digital imaging techniques for quite some time, but its use in diagnostic radiography is relatively new. Digital imaging has expanded so rapidly in the last few years that it has changed forever the way radiographic examinations are viewed.

Although *Digital Radiography and PACS* is intended for entry-level radiography students, we have discovered that few technologists have nearly enough information to allow them to do the best job they can. This book will benefit anyone with the desire to understand why digital imaging works and how they can provide the best imaging techniques possible for better patient care.

As of this writing, we could find no text that pulled together digital imaging and PACs as comprehensively as we have tried to do in this book. All imaging science professionals can benefit not only from reading this book, but also by suggesting updates and improvements. If the information is as forthcoming as we would like, then perhaps among all of us we can get what we need.

REVISIONS TO THIS EDITION

Because digital imaging technology is constantly changing, we have updated our content, particularly in Chapters 4, 5, 6, 7, and 12. In Chapter 4, revisions have been made to the Digitizing the Signal and Speed Class sections. In Chapter 5, revisions have been made to the Imaging Plate Selection, Grid Selection, and Automatic Data Recognition sections. In Chapter 6, the Indirect Conversion, CsI Detectors, Detective Quantum Efficiency, and Spatial Resolution sections have been revised. In Chapter 12, the Quality Control Standards section has been revised.

Keep in mind, however, that if our text does not answer your specific questions or problems, always refer back to your manufacturer's documentation for specific equipment and software functions.

FEATURES

This book was written with the reader in mind; hence, we have attempted to present the information as clearly and simply as possible. We have supplemented textual explanations with as many **illustrations**, **photographs**, and **charts** as would help illuminate ideas without distracting from concepts. Each chapter includes **Objectives** and **Key Terms** lists to help students focus on what they need to learn and finishes with a **Summary** section and **Chapter Review Questions** to reinforce the readings. To ensure a common language, we have included a **Glossary** and an **Abbreviation Table** to completely define key concepts.

ORGANIZATION

Chapter 1 starts with a basic overview of the concepts central to the focus of this book, including latent image formation for both conventional and digital image processing, with an introduction to PACs and how digital image processing integrates with digital storage systems.

Chapter 2 provides a basic overview of the computer, assuming the reader has no prior knowledge or understanding. The chapter introduces basic computer hardware, monitors, operating systems, and computer uses in radiology.

Chapter 3 introduces the reader to computer networking. This chapter covers network classifications, hardware components, and networking topologies. The chapter also introduces the reader to DICOM (digital imaging communication in medicine) and HL-7 (health level 7) to provide a better understanding of digital communication within the radiology department.

Chapter 4 investigates cassette-based digital imaging, with particular attention to how the image is captured, converted, and viewed. Also known as computed radiography (CR), this chapter looks into imaging techniques and equipment necessary to produce CR images.

Chapter 5 looks more deeply into how the cassette-based system functions. Proper selection of imaging factors such as exam menu choices, technical factors, imaging plate size, grids, and markers is discussed as are vendor-driven exposure indicators.

Chapter 6 discusses cassetteless digital imaging and highlights its similarities and differences to cassette-based digital imaging. Both direct and indirect capture methods are discussed, with attention to digital conversion with anamorphous silicon detectors, CCDs, and CSI detectors. We have provided a comparison between detector DQE and that of cassette-based systems, as well as a discussion of the impact of detector size, orientation, and factors that affect spatial resolution.

Chapter 7 takes both cassette-based and cassetteless digital imaging from acquisition to processing, focusing on image histogram formation and automatic rescaling functions. A comparison is made between image latitude in digital imaging and that of conventional film/screen imaging. Contrast enhancement is discussed as are image conversion factors such as the Nyquist theorem, algorithm application, and MTF. Image manipulation factors and image management are also discussed.

Chapter 8 begins the study of Picture Archival and Communication Systems (PACS) with an overview of how a PACS functions and the basic categories of workstations. This chapter covers a simple PACS workflow, showing how the images are moved throughout the department. Also discussed are PACS architectures, common workstation functionality, and several specialty workstation functions.

Chapter 9 introduces the PACS archive. Short-term and long-term archival components are discussed along with their practical uses. Application service providers and disaster recovery are also discussed.

Chapter 10 provides an overview of the following PACS peripherals: film digitizers, film imagers (printers), and CD/DVD burners. Each section provides a basic explanation of operation and their common uses.

Chapter 11 discusses the process of ensuring quality in a PACS. The chapter begins with a basic overview of quality terms and theories. This chapter is dedicated to ensuring display quality, whether it be on monitor or film. Other quality factors are discussed, such as speed, data integrity, and training.

Chapter 12 provides a discussion of total quality theory and includes timelines and schedules for daily, weekly, and monthly quality control activities for the technologist, service personnel, and radiation physicist for cassetteless and cassette-based digital radiography. Repeat analysis, problem reporting, and personal responsibility for proper image marking, repeats, and prevention of artifacts are also discussed.

TEACHING AIDS FOR THE INSTRUCTOR
Instructor's Electronic Resource (IER)
An Instructor's Electronic Resource accompanies the text and resides on Evolve. This resource consists of:

- PowerPoint slides to assist in classroom lecture preparation.
- Test Bank, which includes over 350 questions in Examview format.

- Electronic Image Collection, which includes all the images from the text in PowerPoint and jpeg format.
- Answers to the review questions in the text.

Evolve
Evolve is an interactive learning environment designed to work in coordination with *Digital Radiography and PACS*. Instructors may use Evolve to provide an Internet-based course component that reinforces and expands on the concepts delivered in class.

Evolve may be used to publish the class syllabus, outlines, and lecture notes; set up "virtual office hours" and email communication; share important dates and information through the online class Calendar; and encourage student participation through Chat Rooms and Discussion Boards. Evolve allows instructors to post exams and manage their grade books online. For more information, visit http://evolve.elsevier.com/Carter/digital/ or contact an Elsevier sales representative.

We encourage any correspondence regarding the information contained in this textbook. We will strive to provide the most up-to-date information at the time of publication and we hope that you find this information useful in your classroom and throughout your studies. Please feel free to drop either of us an email with your questions, comments, and suggestions.

Christi E. Carter
Brookhaven College
3939 Valley View Lane
Farmers Branch, TX 75244
ccarter@dcccd.edu

Beth L. Vealé
Midwestern State University
3410 Taft Blvd
Bridwell Hall Room 212
Wichita Falls, TX 76308
beth.veale@mwsu.edu

Acknowledgments

We would like to thank Elsevier for giving us this wonderful opportunity, no matter how painful the process. Christi would also like to thank her family and friends for putting up with her long hours and always lugging around books, papers, and the laptop no matter where she went; her friends and colleagues at Brookhaven College (especially Valerie and Stephanie) for their patience in dealing with her on a day-to-day basis during this process; the Children's Medical Center, Medical Center of Plano, and Trinity Medical Center for allowing her to photograph their departments for this text; and her students for inspiring her to finish this task, knowing that it was really all for them. Beth would like to thank her two reasons for being: Paul and Erin, and her good friends at MSU (Bob, Lynette, Jeff, James, and Gary) for being so supportive and patient. She would especially like to thank the following really special folks: Glenn Hallauer, Carestream; Ralph Schaetzing, Ph.D., Fuji Healthcare (you rock!); John Lampignano and Rees Stuteville who said "Go for it!"; Haley and Corey Smallwood; Kell West Imaging Center; and Excel Imaging. This book is for her students and colleagues who make her want to be a better teacher. Both of us would like to thank Jeanne Olson, Linda Woodard, Luke Held, and David Stein at Elsevier for their support, encouragement, and guidance.

Christi E. Carter, MSRS, RT(R)
Beth L. Vealé, M.Ed., RT(R)(QM)

Contents

DIGITAL RADIOGRAPHY AND PACS

PART I

Introduction

Introduction to Digital Radiography and PACS

1. Define the term digital imaging
2. Explain latent image formation for conventional radiography
3. Describe the latent image formation process for computed radiography
4. Compare and contrast the latent image formation process for indirect capture digital radiography and direct capture digital radiography
5. Explain what a picture archival and communication system (PACS) is and how it is used
6. Define digital imaging and communications in medicine

Computed radiography (CR)
DICOM
Digital imaging
Digital radiography (DR)
Direct capture digital radiography

Indirect capture digital radiography
Picture archival and communication system (PACS)
Teleradiology

This chapter is intended to present a brief overview of digital radiography (DR) (cassette-based and cassette-less systems) and picture archival and communication system (PACS); both topics will be covered in depth in the chapters that follow. The chapter also presents several basic definitions, compares and contrasts digital and analog imaging, and presents the historic development of both DR and PACS. It is important to grasp the basic definitions and concepts before moving to the more involved topics because this information will be useful throughout the textbook.

CONVENTIONAL RADIOGRAPHY

Before defining and discussing digital imaging, a basic understanding of conventional film/screen imaging must be established. Conventional radiography uses film and intensifying screens in its image formation process. Film is placed on one or between two intensifying screens that emit light when struck by x-rays. The light exposes the film in proportion to the amount and energy of the x-rays incident on the screen. The film is then processed with chemicals, and the manifest image appears on the sheet of film. The film is taken to a radiologist and placed on a lightbox for interpretation. For further review of how conventional radiographic images are created, please consult your radiographic imaging textbook for a more in-depth explanation of this process.

DIGITAL IMAGING

Digital imaging is a very broad term. Digital imaging is what allows text, photos, drawings, animations, and video to appear on the World Wide Web. In medicine, digital imaging was first used with the introduction of the computed tomography (CT) scanner by Godfrey Hounsfield in the 1970s. In the decades since then, other imaging modalities have become digital.

The basic definition of **digital imaging** is any imaging acquisition process that produces an electronic image that can be viewed and manipulated on a computer. Most modern medical imaging modalities produce digital images that can be sent through a computer network to a host of locations.

Historical Development of Digital Imaging

Second only to the discovery of the x-ray as a major milestone in medical imaging is the invention of the CT. CT brought about the coupling of the computer and imaging devices. The earliest CT unit built by Hounsfield took several hours to acquire a single slice of information. The machine then took a few days to reconstruct the raw data into a recognizable image. The first commercial CT scanners built were made to image the head only. Figure 1-1 shows one of the early CT scanners built for imaging the head.

Magnetic resonance imaging (MRI) was introduced commercially for health care use in the early 1980s. Several companies began pioneering efforts in the mid to late

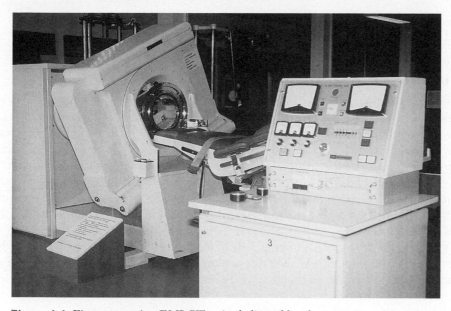

Figure 1-1 First-generation EMI CT unit: dedicated head scanner.
(Photograph taken at Roentgen Museum, Lennep, Germany.)

1970s after the publication of an article by Paul Lauterbur in 1973. Many scientists and researchers were involved in the development of the MRI as we know it today.

Fluoroscopy saw many advances during the 1970s as well thanks to the advances in computer technology. Analog-to-digital converters made it possible to see the dynamic (real-time) image on a television monitor in higher resolution and to store the frames digitally on a computer. Ultrasound and nuclear medicine were easy converts to the digital world early on because the images created in these modalities were simply frame-grabbed (the current image on the screen is captured and sent as an image file) and converted to a digital image. Improved image quality in computed radiography (CR) and digital radiography opened the way for mammography to convert to a digital format.

DIGITAL RADIOGRAPHY

The concept of moving images digitally was by Albert Jutras in Canada during his experimentation with **teleradiology** (moving images via telephone lines to and from remote locations) in the 1950s. Early PACSs were developed by the U.S. military in an effort to move images among Veterans Administration (VA) hospitals and battlefield images to established hospitals. These strides were taking place in the early to mid 1980s, and without the government's participation, this technology would not be where it is today. To provide the PACS a digital image, early analog radiographs were scanned into a computer (digitized) so that the images could be sent from computer to computer. The inherently digital modalities were sent via a PACS first, and then as CR and DR technologies advanced, they joined the digital ranks.

Computed Radiography

Computed radiography, or cassette-based DR, is the digital acquisition modality that uses storage phosphor plates to produce projection images. CR can be used in standard radiographic rooms just like film/screen. The use of CR requires the CR cassettes and phosphor plates, the CR readers (Figure 1-2) and technologist quality control workstation, and a means to view the images, either a printer or a viewing station.

The storage phosphor plates are very similar to our current intensifying screens. The biggest difference is that the storage phosphors can store a portion of the incident x-ray energy in traps within the material for later readout. More will be presented on this topic in Chapter 4.

CR was first introduced commercially in the United States in 1983 by Fuji Medical Systems of Japan (Figure 1-3). The first system consisted of a phosphor storage plate, a reader, and a laser printer to print the image onto film. CR did not take off very quickly

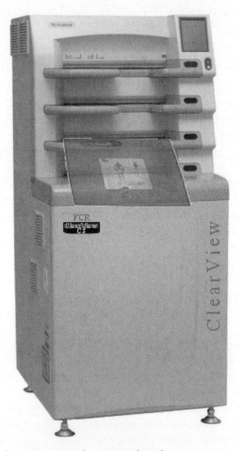

Figure 1-2 Fuji CR reader, cassette and storage-phosphor screen.

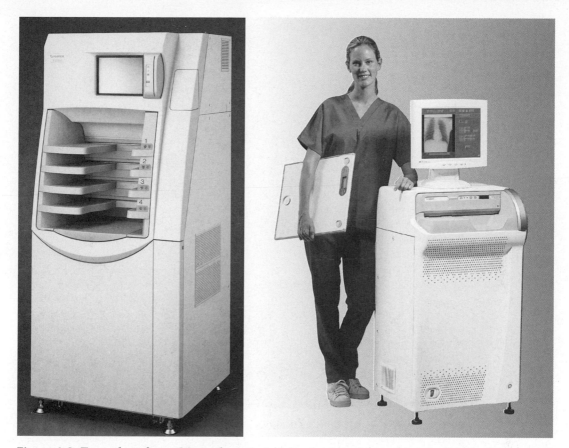

Figure 1-3 Examples of two CR readers. A, A high volume reader capable of processing between 110 and 140 imaging plates per hour. **B,** A much smaller system designed for medical offices, surgery, or intensive care units, capable of processing 50 to 60 imaging plates per hour.
(A, from Ballinger: Merrill's atlas, *ed 10, St. Louis, 2003, Mosby; B, courtesy FujiFilm Medical Systems, USA.)*

because many radiologists were reluctant to embrace the new technology. In the early 1990s, CR began to be installed at a much greater rate because of the technological improvements that had occurred in the decade since its introduction. Several major vendors have CR systems installed in hospitals throughout the United States.

Digital Radiography

Most **digital radiography** (cassette-less) systems use an x-ray absorber material coupled to a flat panel detector or a charged coupled device (CCD) to form the image. Therefore an existing x-ray room needs to be retrofitted with these devices if a new DR room is not installed (Figure 1-4).

DR can be divided into two categories: indirect capture and direct capture. **Indirect capture digital radiography** devices absorb x-rays and convert them into light. The light is then detected by an area-CCD or thin-film transistor (TFT) array and then converted into an electrical signal that is sent to the computer for processing

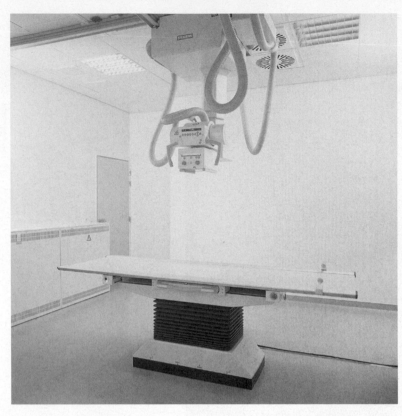

Figure 1-4 Axiom Aristos MX DR unit.
(Courtesy Siemens.)

and viewing (Figure 1-5). Direct capture devices convert the incident x-ray energy directly into an electrical signal, typically using a photoconductor as the x-ray absorber, and send the electrical signal to the computer for processing and viewing (Figure 1-6).

In the early 1970s, several early digital pioneers developed the first clinical application for digital images, digital subtraction angiography (DSA) at the University of Arizona in Tucson. Drs. M. Paul Capp and Sol Nudelman with Hans Roehrig, Dan Fisher, and Meryll Frost developed the precursor to the current full-field DR units. As the technology progressed, several companies began developing large field detectors, first using the CCD technology developed by the military and shortly thereafter using TFT arrays. CCD and TFT technology developed and continues to develop in parallel. Neither technology has proven to be better than the other.

Comparison of CR and DR with Conventional Radiography

When comparing film/screen imaging with CR and DR, several factors should be considered (Table 1-1). For conventional x-ray and CR, a traditional x-ray room with a table and wall Bucky is required. For DR, a detector replaces the Bucky apparatus in both the table and wall stand. Because both conventional radiography and CR use

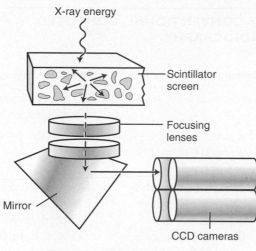

X-ray energy

Scintillator screen

Focusing lenses

Mirror

CCD cameras

CCD Detector with Scintillator Screen

Figure 1-5 The image acquisition process of an indirect capture DR system using CCD technology.

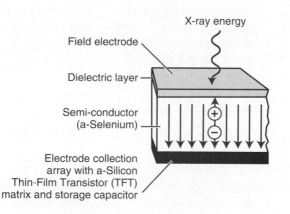
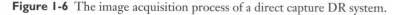

X-ray energy

Field electrode

Dielectric layer

Semi-conductor (a-Selenium)

Electrode collection array with a-Silicon Thin-Film Transistor (TFT) matrix and storage capacitor

Amorphous Selenium DirectRay Dectector

Figure 1-6 The image acquisition process of a direct capture DR system.

cassettes, technologists often rate them the same in terms of ease and efficiency, but DR has an advantage because the processing is done right at the room's console. The image will appear in 3 to 5 seconds, and the technologist knows right away if the image needs to be repeated.

Latent image formation is different with conventional radiography (Figure 1-7), CR, and DR. In conventional radiographic imaging, a film is placed inside a cassette that contains an intensifying screen. When the x-rays strike the intensifying screen, light is produced. The light photons and x-ray photons interact with the silver halide grains in the film emulsion, and an electron is ejected from the halide. The ejected electron is attracted to the sensitivity speck. The speck now has a negative charge, and silver ions are attracted to equal out the charge. This process happens many times

TABLE 1-1   COMPARISON OF CONVENTIONAL, COMPUTED, AND DIGITAL RADIOGRAPHY

Factors Considered	Conventional Radiography	Computed Radiography	Digital Radiography
Imaging room	Traditional x-ray room	Traditional x-ray room	Retrofit traditional x-ray room or install detectors in new room
Ease of use for technologist	Use cassette and film; process with chemicals	Use cassette with phosphor plate; process in CR reader	No cassette; process at console
Latent image formation	X-rays strike intensifying screen; light is emitted, and film exposed to light	X-rays strike phosphor plate. X-ray energy deposited in the phosphor; energy is released from phosphor when stimulated by light in reader	X-rays strike detector. Indirect: phosphor emits light; photodetector (silicon and TFT) detects light and converts to electrical pulse. Direct: X-rays detected by photoconductor and converted to electrical signals
Processing	Image processed by chemicals; image appearance based on technical factors and film/screen combination	Image processed by light; image processing takes place in a quality control station based on preset image algorithms	Image detected; image processing takes place at the acquisition console based on preset image algorithms
Exposure response	Nonlinear; narrow exposure latitude	Linear; wide exposure latitude	Linear; wide exposure latitude
Image contrast	kVp and film response curve	kVp and LUTs	kVp and LUTs
Density	mAs	Image processing LUTs	Image processing LUTs
Scatter radiation	Important for patient dose reduction	Important for patient dose reduction and image processing; the phosphor can be more sensitive to low energy photons	Important for patient dose reduction and image processing; the detector can be more sensitive to low energy photons
Noise	Seen with low mAs and fast screens	Seen with inadequate mAs	Seen with inadequate mAs

within the emulsion to form the latent image. After chemical processing, the sensitivity specks will be processed into black metallic silver, and the manifest image is formed.

In CR, a photostimulable phosphor plate is placed inside the CR cassette. Most storage phosphor plates today are made of a barium fluorohalide (where the halide is bromine and/or iodine) with europium as an activator. When x-rays strike the photo-stimulable phosphor, some light is given off, as in a conventional intensifying screen,

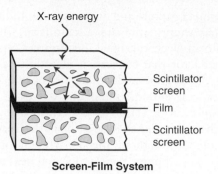

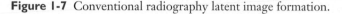

Screen-Film System

Figure 1-7 Conventional radiography latent image formation.

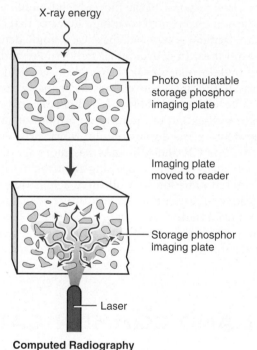

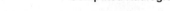

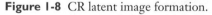

Computed Radiography

Figure 1-8 CR latent image formation.

but some of the photon energy is deposited within the phosphor particles to create the latent image (Figure 1-8). The phosphor plate is then fed through the CR reader. To release the latent image, focused laser light (from one or more lasers) is scanned over the plate, causing the electrons to return to their original state and emitting light in the process. This light is picked up by a photomultiplier tube and converted into an electrical signal. The electrical signal is then sent through an analog-to-digital converter to produce a digital image that can be sent to the technologist review station.

In DR there are no cassettes. The image acquisition device is either built into the table and/or wall stand or enclosed in a portable device. There are two distinct image acquisition methods: indirect capture and direct capture. Indirect capture is very similar to CR in that the x-ray energy stimulates a scintillator, which gives off light that is detected and turned into an electrical signal. With direct capture, the x-ray energy is detected by a photoconductor that converts it directly to a digital electrical signal. This process will be described more in depth in later chapters.

Image processing in conventional radiography is done with chemicals and the shape of the film's response curve. With CR and DR, image processing takes place in a computer. For CR the computer is located near the readers, whether there are several readers distributed throughout the department or there is one centrally located reader. For DR the computer is either located next to the x-ray console or is integrated within the console, and the image is processed before moving on to the next exposure.

The exposure latitude or dynamic range used in conventional radiography is based on the characteristic response of the film, which is nonlinear. Acquiring images with CR or DR, on the other hand, involves using a detector that can respond in a linear manner. The exposure latitude is very wide because a single detector can be sensitive to a wide range of exposures. In conventional radiography, radiographic contrast is primarily controlled by kilovoltage peak (kVp). With CR and DR, kVp still influences subject contrast, but radiographic contrast is primarily controlled by an image processing look-up table. (A look-up table [LUT] is a table that maps the image gray-scale values into some visible output intensity on a monitor or printed film.) With conventional radiography, optical density on film is primarily controlled by milliamperage seconds (mAs). For CR and DR, mAs has more influence on image noise, whereas density is controlled by image processing algorithms (with LUTs). It is important to minimize scattered radiation with all three acquisition systems, but CR and DR can be more sensitive to scatter than screen/film. The materials used in the many CR and DR image acquisition devices are more sensitive to low energy photons. For example, the barium fluorohalide phosphor screens have a k-edge at 37 keV, which produces increased absorption in this energy range, a range that frequently contains x-ray scatter.

PICTURE ARCHIVAL AND COMMUNICATION SYSTEMS

A **picture archival and communication system** is a networked group of computers, servers, and archives that can be used to manage digital images (Figure 1-9). A PACS can accept any image that is in digital imaging and communications in medicine **(DICOM)** format, for which it is set up to receive, whether it is from cardiology, radiology, or pathology. A PACS serves as the fileroom, reading room, duplicator, and courier. It can provide image access to multiple users at the same time, on-demand images, electronic annotation of images, and specialty image processing.

A PACS is often custom designed for a facility. The software is generally the same, but the components are arranged differently. Specific factors are involved in designing a PACS for an institution, such as the volume of patients, the number of areas where

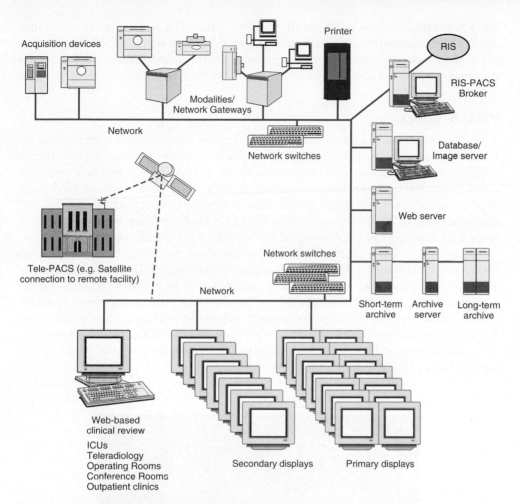

Printer

RIS

Acquisition devices

Modalities/
Network Gateways

Network

RIS-PACS
Broker

Network switches

Database/
Image server

Tele-PACS (e.g. Satellite
connection to remote facility)

Web server

Network switches

Network

Short-term   Archive   Long-term
archive   server   archive

Web-based
clinical review

ICUs
Teleradiology
Operating Rooms
Conference Rooms
Outpatient clinics

Secondary displays   Primary displays

Figure 1-9 PACS network.

images are interpreted, the locations where images are viewed by physicians other than radiologists, and the money available for purchase.

In the mid to early 1980s, different versions of PACS were being developed, primarily by research and academic institutions. They were homegrown and usually involved one or possibly two modalities. These early systems were hard to put together because there was little standardization in image formats. Each vendor had its own proprietary way of archiving images, and there was little need or desire to share archiving methods. Once DICOM (standards that allow imaging modalities and PACS to communicate in the same "language") was established, more vendors began using it to communicate between modalities and PACS. Full-scale acceptance of DICOM was pushed by the consumer to make it possible for equipment from different manufacturers to talk to each other. The first full-scale PACS in the United States was installed at the VA Medical Center in Baltimore in 1993. Their PACS covered all modalities except mammography. Soon after installing their PACS, the Baltimore Medical Center asked the vendor to interface to their radiology information system (RIS), hospital information system (HIS), and electronic medical record (EMR).

PACS Uses

A PACS is made up of many different parts, such as the reading stations, physician review stations, web-access, technologist quality control stations, administrative stations, archive systems, and many interfaces to various hospital and radiology systems. Early PACSs were mainly seen in radiology and sometimes in cardiology departments. Now a PACS can receive images from any department in the hospital that sends in a DICOM format for which the PACS has been set up to receive. Archive space (and expense) can now be shared among different hospital departments.

Many PACS reading stations also have image processing capabilities. Radiologists can remain at their workstation and do three-dimensional (3D) reconstructions of a CT (Figure 1-10) or stitch a complete spine together to perform specialized measurement functions for scoliosis. Some PACSs also offer orthopedic workstations for orthopedic surgeons to plan joint replacement surgery before beginning the operation. Specialized software allows the surgeon to load a plain x-ray of the joint and a template for the replacement joint and to match the best replacement to the patient. This software saves a great deal of time in the operating room.

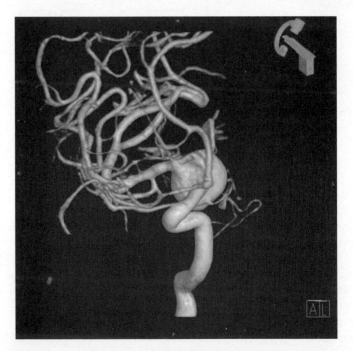

Figure 1-10 Three-dimensional reconstruction of an aneurysm. *(Courtesy Siemens.)*

SUMMARY

All of the topics covered in this chapter will be covered in depth more throughout the book. In summary:

- Digital imaging is any imaging acquisition process that produces an electronic image that can be viewed and manipulated on a computer.
- CR is the digital acquisition modality that uses photostimulable phosphor plates to produce digital projection images.
- DR is divided into two categories: indirect capture and direct capture.
- Indirect capture uses a detector that produces light when struck by x-rays, and then the light is captured and converted to an electrical signal.
- Direct capture uses a detector that captures the x-ray energy and converts it directly to an electrical signal.
- A PACS is a networked group of computers, servers, and archives that can be used to manage digital images.
- DICOM is a standard that allows imaging modalities and PACSs to communicate in the same "language."
- PACSs are made up of many different parts, such as the reading stations, physician review stations, web-access, technologist quality control stations, administrative stations, archive systems, and many interfaces to various hospital and radiology systems.

CHAPTER REVIEW QUESTIONS

1. Define digital imaging.

2. What is the latent image formation for conventional imaging?

3. Compare the latent image formation for conventional imaging with cassette-based digital radiography.

4. How is the latent image formed when using cassette-less digital radiography?

5. What does the acronym PACS stand for, and what are its uses?

6. What does the acronym DICOM stand for, and how is it used?

Basic Principles

CHAPTER 2

Basic Computer Principles

1. Describe the major components of a computer
2. Define binary code, bit, and byte, and discuss how they relate to one another
3. List and define the hardware components discussed in this chapter
4. List the three most common types of monitors
5. Explain the measurements used to classify monitors
6. Compare and contrast an operating system and application software
7. Discuss the uses of computers in a radiology department

KEY TERMS

Aspect ratio
Binary code
Basic input/output system (BIOS)
Bit
Bus
Byte
Central processing unit (CPU)
Complementary metal oxide semiconductor (CMOS)
Computer
Dot pitch

Hard drive
Matrix
Memory
Motherboard
Operating system (OS)
Pixel
Port
Power supply
Refresh rate
Resolution
Viewable area

A **computer** is a programmable electronic device that can store, retrieve, and process data. This chapter will provide an overview of how a computer works, the basic hardware components of a computer system, the differences between each type of system, and the different types of monitors. These topics will be explored to provide a basic overview of computers so that picture archival and communication (PAC) and digital radiographic systems can be better understood in the following chapters.

HOW DOES THE COMPUTER WORK?

In its basic form, a computer consists of input, output, and processing devices (Figure 2-1). Input devices are keyboards, mice, microphones, barcode readers, touch screens, and image scanners, and any of these can be found in any modern radiology department. Common output devices are monitors, printers, and speakers. The computer also has various communication devices that it uses to share information. The processing of information is done in the central processing unit (CPU), which will be detailed later in the chapter.

    The computer takes data from the user and processes it using a machine language of 1s and 0s, known as **binary code.** The computer processing is performed by a series of transistors, which are switches that are either on or off (Figure 2-2). If the transistor circuit is closed and current passes through, it is assigned a value of 1. If no current passes because of the circuit being open, it is assigned a value of 0. A computer's transistors can be switched on and off millions of times in a second. Each 1 and 0 represents a bit. A **bit** is a single unit of data. A **byte** is made up of eight bits and is the amount of memory needed to store one alphanumeric character (Figure 2-3). Because one character takes up a byte of memory, memory is generally talked about in kilobytes, megabytes, gigabytes, and even terabytes.

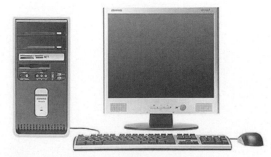

Figure 2-1 A basic personal computer consisting of a CPU, keyboard, mouse, and LCD monitor.

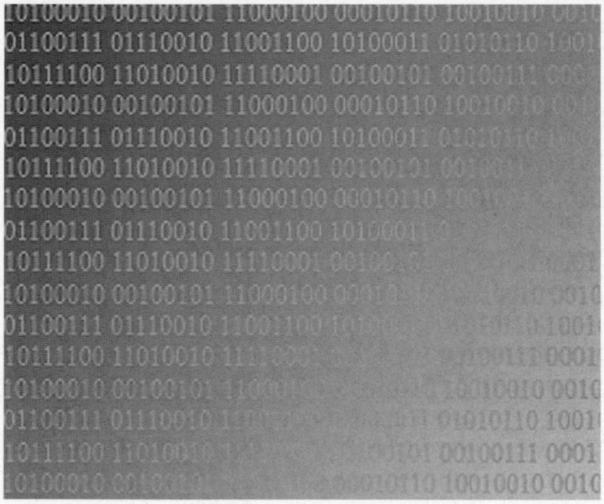

Figure 2-2 Binary code consists of 1s and 0s.

HARDWARE COMPONENTS

"The Box"

The computer encasement is made from a heavy metal and has two major functions:

1. To hold all of the components in a relatively cool, clean, and safe environment
2. To shield the outside environment from the radio frequencies being emitted by the electronic components of the computer

The box comes in two major configurations: the desktop model and the tower (Figure 2-4). The desktop model is generally positioned in a horizontal box, whereas a tower model is in a vertical box. As the name implies, most desktop models are placed on the desk underneath the monitor. The tower model is generally placed underneath the desk within arm's reach of the operator. The biggest disadvantage of the desktop model is the space it takes up on the desk; the smaller the box, the less room for expansion and upgrades. The tower model consistently provides adequate room for expansion of components, and it is easily placed out of the way and off the work surface.

The Motherboard

The **motherboard** (Figure 2-5) is the largest circuitry board inside the computer, and it contains many important small components to make the computer function properly. This chapter will only cover a few of these components in detail: the CPU, basic input/output system (BIOS), memory, bus, ports, and complementary metal oxide semiconductor (CMOS).

Letter	Binary code
A	01000001
B	01000010
C	01000011
D	01000100
E	01000101
F	01000110
G	01000111
H	01001000
I	01001001
J	01001010
K	01001011
L	01001100
M	01001101
N	01001110
O	01001111
P	01010000
Q	01010001
R	01010010
S	01010011
T	01010100
U	01010101
V	01010110
W	01010111
X	01011000
Y	01011001
Z	01011010

Letter	Binary code
a	01100001
b	01100010
c	01100011
d	01100100
e	01100101
f	01100110
g	01100111
h	01101000
i	01101001
j	01101010
k	01101011
l	01101100
m	01101101
n	01101110
o	01101111
p	01110000
q	01110001
r	01110010
s	01110011
t	01110100
u	01110101
v	01110110
w	01110111
x	01111000
y	01111001
z	01111010

Figure 2-3 Binary representation of the alphabet.

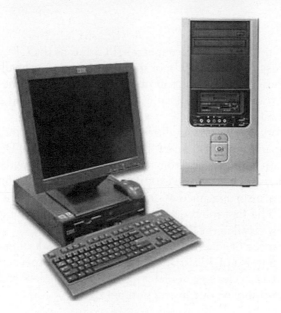

Figure 2-4 The desktop model is pictured on the left, and the tower is pictured on the right.

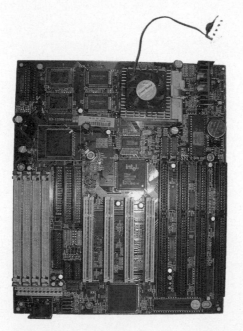

Figure 2-5 Motherboard.

The CPU

Many people refer to the personal computer's (PC) box as the CPU. This is incorrect. The **central processing unit (CPU),** or microprocessor, is a small chip found on the motherboard (Figure 2-6). The microprocessor is the brain of the computer. It consists of a series of transistors (discussed earlier) that are arranged to manipulate data received from the software.

Microprocessors come in many different sizes and speeds and are manufactured by two major companies, Intel (Figure 2-7) and Advanced Micro Devices (AMD). The CPU's basic tasks are to read data from storage, manipulate the data, and then move the data back to storage or send it to external devices, such as monitors or printers.

The microprocessor is named after its manufacturer and the speed at which it manipulates data. The first microprocessor to be placed in a computer was made in 1979 by Intel and was called the 8088.

It had a clock speed of a mere 4.77 MHz. The more modern Pentium 4 microprocessor has speeds upward of 3.2 to 3.8 GHz. To put these speeds in perspective, the 8088 needed about 12 cycles to complete one basic instruction, and the modern Pentium processor can complete one instruction per cycle.

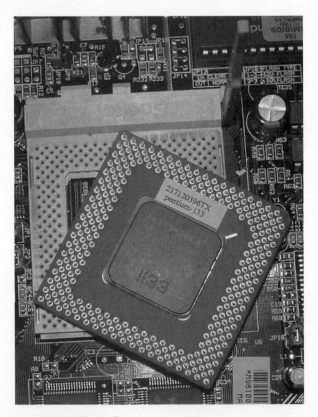

Figure 2-6 Central processing unit.

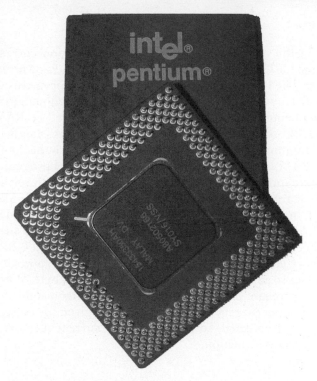

Figure 2-7 An Intel Pentium processor.

The BIOS

The **basic input/output system (BIOS)** contains a simple set of instructions for the computer. The microprocessor uses the BIOS during the boot-up process of the computer to help bring the computer to life. The BIOS also runs the start-up diagnostics on the system to make sure all of the peripherals are functioning properly. After the computer has booted up, the BIOS oversees the basic functions of receiving and interpreting signals from the keyboard and interchanging information with various ports. The BIOS is the intermediary between the operating system (OS) and the hardware.

The Bus

The **bus** is a series of connections, controllers, and chips that creates the information highway of the computer. There are several buses throughout the computer that connect the microprocessor, the system memory, and various peripherals. Most modern PCs have what is called a peripheral component interconnect (PCI) bus on the motherboard to serve as the connection of information to the various adapters. Other buses found within the computer are for the small computer system interface (SCSI) connections, the accelerated graphics port (AGP) for video adapters, and the universal serial bus (USB) for a variety of devices. Simply put, the bus provides the connections for the information to flow within the computer.

Memory

The **memory** in the computer is used to store information currently being processed within the CPU (Figure 2-8). This memory is also known as random access memory (RAM). The RAM is short-term storage for open programs. The microprocessor has a small amount of memory within itself but not enough to tackle the large amounts of data being generated by high-level programs. The RAM will take the data from the CPU so that the CPU can handle the processing needs of the programs that are running. The RAM is only temporary; once the computer has been turned off, the RAM is wiped clean. With today's high level programs and graphics, computers require more memory to function at an acceptable level. There are many different types of RAM available: DRAM, EDO RAM, VRAM, SRAM, SDRAM, SIMM, DIMM, and ECO. Most modern PCs have an SDRAM-DDR, but some may have RDRAM for high graphics programs. Memory is measured in bytes and can be found in configurations such as 128 MB, 512 MB, and 1 GB. In some of the first PCs, memory came in 16-kilobyte blocks and sold for approximately 100 dollars, which equates to approximately 4000 dollars per megabyte. With more modern pricing, one can purchase 256 MB of SDRAM for approximately 30 dollars, which equates to 12 cents per megabyte. These figures are given for perspective purposes and become quickly outdated, so please research current memory capacities and prices for up-to-date information.

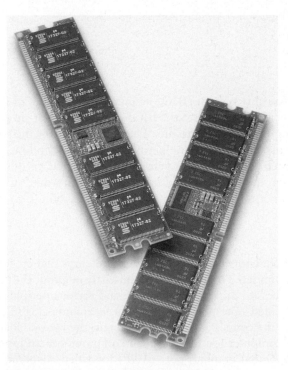

Figure 2-8 Memory chip.
(Courtesy Sun Corporation.)

Ports

The computer's **ports** are a collection of connectors sticking out of the back of the PC that link adapter cards, drives, printers, scanners, keyboards, mice, and other peripherals that may be used. There are many different types of ports, such as parallel, serial, USB, integrated drive electronics (IDE), and SCSI. We will take a look at each of these types and how they may be used within a system.

A parallel port is a 25-pin connector found on the back of most modern PCs (Figure 2-9). The parallel port is synonymous with a printer port because it is most often used for this purpose. A parallel port can send 8 bits of data through the connection, whereas a serial port can only send 1 bit of data down a single wire. A serial port can be universally used for many of the components plugged into the computer, such as a mouse, which does not require the speed of a parallel port. Most serial ports are of the 9-pin variety, but some can have up to 25-pin connectors.

USBs are a common interface connection used between most devices commonly used today (Figure 2-10). The advantage of a USB port is that multiple devices may be

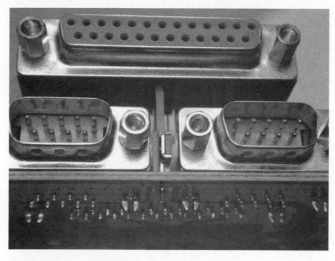

Figure 2-9 Parallel port.

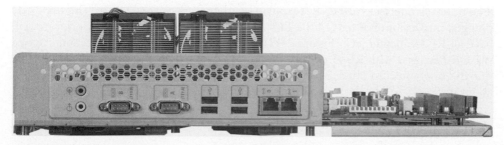

Figure 2-10 USB port.
(Courtesy Sun Corporation.)

connected into one port. In older computers there were only ports for the keyboard and the mouse, one parallel port for a printer, and one serial port for a modem. By using USB ports the user can connect up to 127 devices to one single USB port. Most computers have more than one USB port available, so the possible connections are many.

IDE ports can be found on the motherboard and connect the hard drive, floppy drive, and CD-ROM drive to the board. A series of ribbon cable runs throughout the computer to connect the IDE devices to the IDE port on the motherboard. The fifth type of port is the SCSI port. It is the fastest and most versatile way for a PC to communicate with its peripherals. A single SCSI controller can manage up to seven devices through a daisy chain connection. The most common SCSI devices are hard drives, CD-ROM drives, scanners, and printers.

CMOS

The **complementary metal oxide semiconductor (CMOS)** is a special type of memory chip that uses a small rechargeable or lithium battery to retain information about the PC's hardware while the computer is turned off. The CMOS is also the location of the system clock that keeps track of the date and time. The system clock uses a vibrating quartz crystal to set the speed for the CPU. A single tick of the clock represents the time it takes to turn a transistor on and off. Because modern CPUs are measured in gigahertz, a PC with a 3.0-GHz CPU would have a system clock that would tick 3 billion times per second. Any changes in the system after the last basic system configuration will be detected, and the system will be prompted to install the new hardware.

Sound Card

The sound card contains all of the circuitry for recording and reproducing sound on the PC. It may be in the form of an expansion card, or it may be built into several chips found on the motherboard. Ports are located externally to connect amplified speakers, headphones, microphone, and a compact disk (CD) player input into the computer. The sound card interprets many different file types such as waveform audio (WAV) files, moving picture experts group audio layer 3 (MP3) files, and musical instrument digital interface (MIDI) files.

Network Card

The network interface card (NIC) can come either as an expansion card (Figure 2-11) plugged into a slot or as part of the PC motherboard circuitry. The network card will have an RJ-45 adapter jack (Figure 2-12) at the rear of the PC for the acceptance of a twisted-pair wire with RJ-45 connector (Figure 2-13). This network card will enable this PC to connect to other PCs that are on the same network. Detailed information about networks will be discussed in the next chapter.

Power Supply

The **power supply** (Figure 2-14) delivers all electricity to the PC and contains a fan to help keep the inside of the computer cool. It contains a transformer that converts

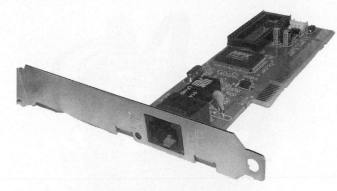

Figure 2-11 Network interface card (NIC).

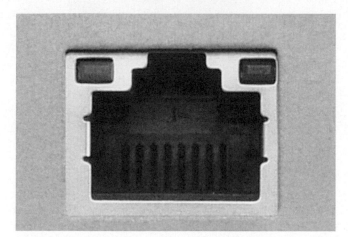

Figure 2-12 RJ-45 jack.

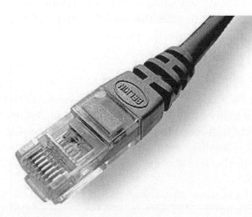

Figure 2-13 RJ-45 connector.

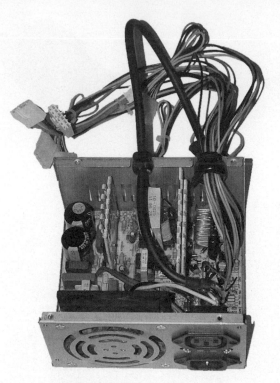

Figure 2-14 Power supply.

the wall outlet alternating current (AC) to direct current (DC) in the voltages appropriate for each powered device. All components, from the motherboard to the hard drive, get their power directly from the main supply through different colored wires that end in plastic shielded connectors. The power supplies deliver +/– 12 V, +/– 5 V, and in some machines +3.3 V. Power supplies are rated in watts. Most power supplies deliver between 150 to 300 W, but some computers require a 400-W power supply. The power supply is designed to take the brunt of the force if the computer ever receives a power surge. In such a case, the power supply is easily replaced.

Hard Drive

The **hard drive** is the main repository for programs and documents on a PC. The hard drive is made up of many hard, thin magnetic platters that are stacked one on top of the other with only enough space for a read-write head to glide over the surface of the disks (Figure 2-15). The disks are spun at a fast speed by a small motor, and the read/write head glides to the area that houses the particular information needed and reads or writes as asked.

The early disks had a storage capacity of 10 MB and could be accessed in approximately 80 ms. The more modern disks can hold upward of 100 GB with an access speed of 8.7 ms. As storage capacity has skyrocketed, the price per megabyte of storage

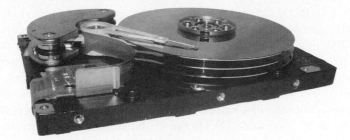

Figure 2-15 Looking inside the hard drive.

has drastically decreased. The drives may be faster than ever, but they are still the slowest part of the PC because they are both mechanical and electrical. These figures were given for perspective purposes and become quickly outdated, so please research current hard drive capacities and prices.

CD/DVD Drive

A CD is a thin injection-molded polycarbonate plastic disk (Figure 2-16). The disk is impressed from a mold to form microscopic bumps that indicate either a 1 or 0 to the computer. Over the bumps is a reflective layer of aluminum, and over that is a clear protective coat of acrylic. A CD can hold up to 74 minutes of music or approximately 780 MB of data.

A digital versatile disk (DVD) holds up to seven times more than the CD, which equates to about 9.4 (single-sided) to 17 GB (double-sided) of data. A DVD has multiple layers of polycarbonate plastic. Aluminum is used behind the inner layers, and gold is used behind the outer layers. The gold is semireflective so that it allows the laser to penetrate through to the inner layers of plastic.

There are three main types of CD/DVD drives available in today's market: the ROM (read-only memory), the R (write once–read many), and the RW (read and write

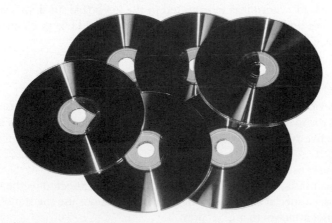

Figure 2-16 Compact disks.

many times). CD-ROM drives were placed into early computers. Few computers today can be bought with a simple ROM drive installed. Most modern computers have either a CD-RW or a CD/DVD-RW. With an R or RW drive, information that needs to be saved, transported, or archived can be "burned" (information written on a disk). The information is burned onto the disk, starting in the center and spiraling out to the edge of the disk. The laser burns a tiny depression (pit) into the disk to represent the data being saved. A burned disk will be a series of pits and lands, or areas that were not burned by the laser. Two-sided DVDs can be burned on both sides to double the capacity of the disk.

How CD/DVD Drives Work

A CD/DVD drive is found on the front of the encasement of a computer. The drive consists of a disk tray, a motor, a read head, and possibly a write head. The drive has a small door that opens horizontally, and a tray appears for the disk to be placed. After the door closes, a motor constantly varies the speed of the disk so that the portion above the read head spins at a constant speed no matter its location over the disk. The laser beam of the read head penetrates the disk and strikes the reflective layer. If the laser strikes a land area, the light reflects back; if the laser strikes a pit, the light is scattered. The light reflected back is read by a light-sensing diode that translates the impulses into 1s and 0s for the computer to generate into recognizable data.

Peripherals

Keyboard

There are two basic types of keyboards: soft and click. If there is an audible sound when the keys are depressed, it is a click keyboard. The first keyboards made by IBM were click keyboards. Most modern keyboards connect using an IBM programming system 2 (PS/2) connection and connect into the back of the box. Some keyboards use the USB connection because of its versatility and ease of use. With the advent of wireless connections, keyboard makers use either infrared or radio frequency (RF) signals.

When the keys are depressed on the keyboard, a signal is sent through the switch to the motherboard, where it is interpreted in the keyboard microprocessor. Because of all the switches underneath the keys, keyboards should be kept clean, and food and drink should never be consumed near the keyboard.

Mouse

A mouse is a device with two or sometimes three buttons that allow the user to move the computer's cursor to activate and perform functions within the computer's software.

There are five types of mouse connections (all are serial-type connections):

- Serial mouse: uses a standard serial connection
- Bus mouse: uses a dedicated controller card that is connected to the motherboard
- PS/2 mouse: a special connection for mice that does not use the standard serial port
- USB mouse: attaches to a USB port
- Infrared mouse: uses the computer's infrared port (wireless)

There are three types of mice commonly used:

- Mechanical: This mouse uses a hard rubber ball inside an opening on the bottom that is surrounded by sensing devices. The ball moves around based on the movement of the user's hand over the mouse and triggers the sensors within the mouse to move the cursor on the screen.
- Optical: This mouse has a high-intensity diode that bounces light off surfaces and back to a receiver inside the mouse. As with the mechanical mouse, the cursor is made to move by the movements of the mouse over a hard surface and by the light that is reflected back to the sensors within the mouse.
- Optomechanical: This mouse is a hybrid of mechanical and optical mouse. It uses a rubber ball that interacts with rollers that trigger the optical sensors within the mouse. Light is reflected back to the sensors based on the movement of the rollers.

Scanners

Scanners are devices that capture drawings or written paper documents and convert them into a digital image or document that can be edited. Special image scanners in radiology departments are used to convert an analog (film) image into a digital image. The purpose is to provide a way to compare a hardcopy image with a digital image on a PAC system (PACS). More information will be given on this topic in Chapter 10.

Speakers

Speakers receive sound data from a sound card that is either built into the motherboard or is an expansion card. The sound data are converted from an electrical signal to a series of vibrations in the speaker to create sound. Speakers have become an integral part of the modern PC because they give audible signals from the software to alert us to various tasks.

Microphones

Microphones are used to record voice or to use voice dictation software. Voice dictation software is becoming more common in radiology departments. The technology has progressed to a point that most people's voices can be recognized by the system's software.

MONITORS

There are two major types of monitors: the cathode ray tube (CRT) and the liquid crystal display (LCD); a third type, the plasma screen, is quickly gaining acceptance. To understand how these monitors work, we must first look at several basic terms and measurements related to onscreen viewing.

A basic picture element on a display is known as a **pixel.** A pixel is an individual controllable set of dot triads. A dot triad is a grouping of one red dot, one green dot, and one blue dot. The number of pixels on a display is known as its **resolution.** The more pixels in an image, the higher the resolution of the image and the more information that can be displayed. Resolution can also be defined as the process or capability of distinguishing between individual parts of an image that are adjacent. Pixels are arranged in a **matrix,** a rectangular or square table of numbers that represents the pixel intensity to be displayed on the monitor. Common screen resolutions are 1024×768, 1280×1024, 2048×1536, and 2048×2560. The last two matrices are common in image viewing applications.

A third measurement is dot pitch. **Dot pitch** is the measurement of how close the dots are located to one another within a pixel; the smaller the dot pitch of a display, the finer the resolution. Dot pitch may be expressed as aperture grille pitch or slot pitch, depending on the monitor maker.

One of the most important measurements of a monitor is its refresh rate or vertical scanning rate. The **refresh rate** is the measure of how fast the monitor rewrites the screen or the number of times that the image is redrawn on the display each second. The refresh rate helps to control the flicker seen by the user; the higher the refresh rate, the less flicker. Most refresh rates on today's computers are set between 60 and 75 Hz; the image is redrawn 60 to 75 times per second. Another set of display terms is aspect ratio and viewable area. The **aspect ratio** is the ratio of the width of the monitor to the height of the monitor. Most CRT monitors have an aspect ratio of 4:3; LCD monitors have a ratio of 16:9. The **viewable area** is measured diagonally from one corner of the display to the opposite corner.

CRT

The CRT monitors are the most popular monitors on the market (Figure 2-17). The CRT consists of a cathode and anode within a vacuum tube. The CRT works much like an x-ray tube, in that the cathode boils off a cloud of electrons and then a potential difference is placed on the tube. A stream of electrons is sent across to the monitor's anode, which is a sheet of glass coated with a phosphor layer. The electrons strike the phosphor on the glass, causing the glass to emit a color, which is determined by the intensity of the interaction and area with which the electrons interacted.

The electrons interact with either a red, green, or blue dot to form the color and image that is being sent from the video card signal. The electron beam starts in the upper left corner and scans across the glass from side to side and top to bottom, and once it reaches the bottom, it starts back over at the top left. On average, most monitors have 350 lines to be scanned. Earlier we discussed the refresh rate being 60 to 75 Hz. This equates to 350 lines being scanned 60 to 75 times per second.

LCD

An LCD monitor produces images by shining or reflecting light through a layer of liquid crystal and a series of color filters (Figure 2-18). An LCD has two pieces of polarized glass with a liquid crystal material between the two. Light is allowed through the first layer of glass, and when a current is applied to the liquid crystal, it aligns and allows light in varying intensities through to the next layer of glass through color filters to form the colors and images seen on the display.

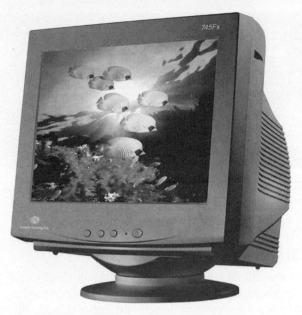

Figure 2-17 Cathode ray tube (CRT) monitor.

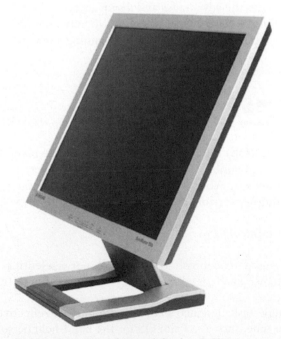

Figure 2-18 Liquid crystal display (LCD).

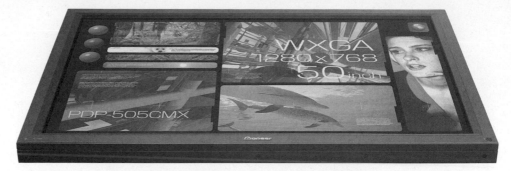

Figure 2-19 Plasma display.
(Courtesy Pioneer Inc.)

Plasma Displays

Plasma displays are still new to the consumer market (Figure 2-19). They have been heavily used in government and military applications since the late 1960s. The plasma displays are made up of many small fluorescent lights that are illuminated to form the color of the image. The plasma display varies the intensities of the various light combinations to produce a full range of color.

Monitor Advantages and Disadvantages

Most consumers want a monitor that can provide the highest resolution for the best price. Table 2-1 outlines the advantages and disadvantages of the three major types of monitors. Most radiology departments have traditionally used the CRT because of its superior resolution, but LCDs are increasingly gaining popularity because they are slimmer and lighter.

OPERATING SYSTEMS

An **operating system (OS)** is the software that controls the computer hardware and acts as a bridge between applications and the hardware. There are three major OSs in use today: Windows by Microsoft, the Macintosh OS, and UNIX/Linux. PCs generally run a Windows version of an OS, such as Windows 95, 98, 2000, ME, XP, or NT.

There are four types of OSs:

- Real-time OS: used to control specific machinery, scientific instruments, and industrial systems, such as digital x-ray consoles found on modern x-ray equipment.
- Single-user, single-task: designed so that a computer can effectively do one task for one person at a time, such as a Palm OS for the hand-held personal organizer.

TABLE 2-1   ADVANTAGES AND DISADVANTAGES OF CRT, LCD, AND PLASMA MONITORS

Monitor Type	Advantages	Disadvantages
CRT	Less expensive	Bulky
	Better color representation	The larger the viewing area, the deeper and heavier the unit
	More responsive than LCD	Not easily adjusted for viewing at different heights and angles
	Can provide multiple resolutions	
	More rugged and can sustain rough handling	
LCD	Takes up less space than a CRT	Costs more than CRT
	Consumes less power than CRT	Less of a viewing angle
	Produces less heat than CRT	Not as bright as CRT
	Surface produces little or no glare	Each display is only capable of working with one physical resolution
	Requires a smaller frame around display	
Plasma	Wide screen with a thin depth	High cost
	Brighter than LCD	Low availability
	Can be viewed at varying angles	
	Light weight	

- Single-user, multitask: designed for one user to perform multiple functions at the same time, such as the OS on a PC.
- Multiuser: designed to handle multiple users and multiple tasks at the same time, such as UNIX running on a large server or as a mainframe computer supporting an entire company.

The computer must have an OS for it to be able to fully come up and function as it was intended. The OS takes over just after the computer wakes up and allows the computer to begin doing tasks. All other software run using the OS. The various programs that are used on the computer are specifically designed to run on the OS that is loaded on the computer. Early OSs, such as Microsoft–Disk Operating System (MS-DOS), were command based and very difficult to use. The user needed to know word commands to type in to get the computer to do simple tasks, such as saving a file. Today most computers use what is called graphical user interface (GUI) to perform various computer functions. A GUI (goo-ee) is a picture (icon)-based program, where the mouse is used to point and click on the function that needs to be performed. The GUI also has easy to use drop-down word menus that can be selected to perform various functions.

As mentioned earlier, IBM-type PCs have traditionally used a Windows-based OS. Large workstations that are used to complete multiple tasks may use Windows NT, or they may opt to use UNIX or Linux for the OS. UNIX is a very robust OS. It was first developed by Bell Laboratories and was given out free to universities. It is primarily used by industry for larger server applications. Some PACS vendors began their software on UNIX-based systems but have since migrated to the Windows platform because of cost, ease of use, and customer demand. Linux was derived from UNIX by a Finnish computer science student and is widely used by computer aficionados. Linux is what is known as open-source software; programmers can make changes in the code as long as the changes are shared with others.

All digital medical imaging devices have some sort of OS running behind the user interface. Depending on the vendor, it may be one of the three discussed here or it may be a proprietary (written and known only by the vendor) system developed specifically for a particular device. PACS is no exception. Most modern PACSs use a Windows-based platform, but some may still use UNIX on their large servers because of its exceptional multitasking capabilities.

COMPUTERS IN THE RADIOLOGY DEPARTMENT

Computers are used throughout radiology departments, from the front desk to the file room and from the technologist's work area to the radiologist's reading room. Many computer applications are used throughout the day by the various staff within the department to improve the care that is given to the patient. In most areas, a simple computer can do the job, but in some more robust applications, a specialty workstation is needed to handle the complicated tasks. Most radiology imaging equipment manufactured today has a computer built into the machine itself, or it has a separate computer that is attached for various applications.

Computer hardware and software are chosen to match the applications used by the staff. Comfort, cost, quality, and purpose are just four areas that are addressed when choosing the appropriate equipment and accessories. For example, a radiologist would require a monitor with high brightness, high resolution, and a large screen to view digital images for diagnosis, whereas a file room clerk would only need a basic monitor.

SUMMARY

- A computer is a programmable electronic device that can store, retrieve, and process data.
- A bit is a single unit of data. There are 8 bits in a byte.
- A computer consists of input, output, and processing devices.
- Input = keyboard, mouse, scanner, barcode reader, and microphone
- Output = monitor, printer, and speakers
- Processing = motherboard, microprocessor, BIOS, bus, memory, ports, and CMOS

- Modern computers contain many types of drives: hard drives, CD-ROM, CD-R, CD-RW, DVD-R, DVD-RW, and floppy. These drives perform specific tasks and functions for the computer.
- Various expansion cards are used within modern PCs: sound cards, network cards, and other peripheral cards.
- Keyboards and mice are the most common input devices. There are various types of each.
- Monitors are measured by several factors: resolution, dot pitch, refresh rate, aspect ratio, and viewable area.
- There are three types of monitors: CRT, LCD, and plasma.
- An OS is the software that controls the computer hardware and acts as a bridge between applications and hardware.
- Computers are found throughout the radiology department, and each has been chosen to fulfill a specific purpose.

CHAPTER REVIEW QUESTIONS

1. What is a computer?

2. Define binary code, bit, and byte.

3. Name several computer hardware components, and list their uses.

4. What are the three major types of monitors, and what are their advantages and disadvantages?

5. What are the measurements used to classify monitor quality?

6. Name and define the different types of OSs.

7. How are computers utilized in the radiology department?

CHAPTER 3

Networking and Communication Basics

1. Distinguish between different types of networks (geographic and component roles)
2. Identify common network hardware components
3. Describe different types of network cabling and their uses
4. Define network communication protocol
5. Differentiate between the common network topologies
6. Discuss the use of DICOM in medical imaging
7. Define HL-7, and describe its use in health care information systems

KEY TERMS

Bus topology
Client-based network
Coaxial cable
Digital imaging and communications in medicine (DICOM)
Fiberoptic cable
HL-7
Hospital information system
Local area network (LAN)
Mesh topology
Network
Network bridge
Network hub
Network interface card (NIC)
Network protocol

Network router
Network switch
Peer-to-peer network
Radiology information system
Ring topology
Server
Server-based network
Star topology
Thick-client
Thin-client
Topology
Twisted-pair wire
Wide area network (WAN)
Wireless
Wireless access point

People use all types of networks every day to do things like check the status of a package being shipped or register for a class at school. Many daily tasks involve transferring information, either from person to person (Figure 3-1) or from computer to computer (Figure 3-2).

A computer **network** is defined as (1) two or more objects sharing resources and information, or (2) computers, terminals, and servers that are interconnected by communication channels sharing data and program resources. Devices other than computers can also be found on a network, such as printers, scanners, and barcode readers.

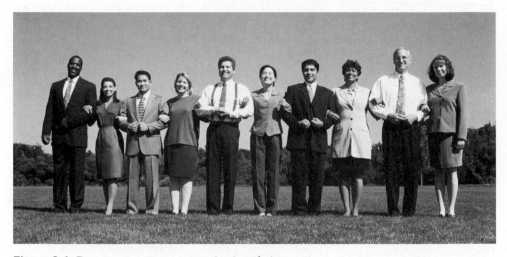

Figure 3-1 Person-to-person communication chain.

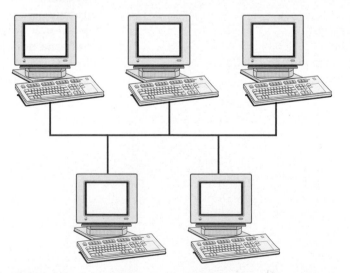

Figure 3-2 Five computers connected via a network to share resources.

These devices can be shared among a group of computers to save money and space for the users.

This chapter explores network classifications, whether they are based on geographic boundaries or the various roles that the hardware components play. An overview of the basic hardware components that make up a computer network and how the networks are physically constructed is also included. This chapter also provides a brief introduction to how medical devices, such as computed tomography (CT) scanners and computed radiography (CR) readers, fit within a network and how they communicate.

NETWORK CLASSIFICATIONS

Geographic Classifications

A network can be classified into two major geographic categories: local area network (LAN) and wide area network (WAN). (Other geographic classifications exist but are of little consequence to radiology.) These two terms are fairly self-explanatory: a LAN is close by, whereas a WAN expands over a distance.

LAN

A **local area network (LAN)** (Figure 3-3) is a small area networked with a series of cables or wireless access points that allow computers to share information and devices on the same network. These are the least expensive to install, and they are much faster than a WAN because of their smaller size. A LAN has the fastest communication technology because less equipment and fewer resources are needed to complete the network. Generally the larger networks are composed of several LANs interconnected to create the WANs. The picture archival and communication system (PACS) workstations in a radiology reading room would be considered a LAN. The computers are interconnected and communicate by sharing images and reports.

WAN

A **wide area network (WAN)** (Figure 3-4) is a network that spans a large area: city, state, nation, continent, or the world. It is used to connect computers that are not physically attached through conventional network cables but are rather connected through other means, such as telephone lines, satellite links, or other types of communication cable. The use of these long distance communication links drives up the operating costs of this type of network because most often these communication links are owned by a separate company, and because of the distance covered, the cost of having the highest speed equipment is expensive.

Component Role Classification

Networks are typically classified as either peer-to-peer or server/client-based, depending on what role their various components play. The network is classified according to

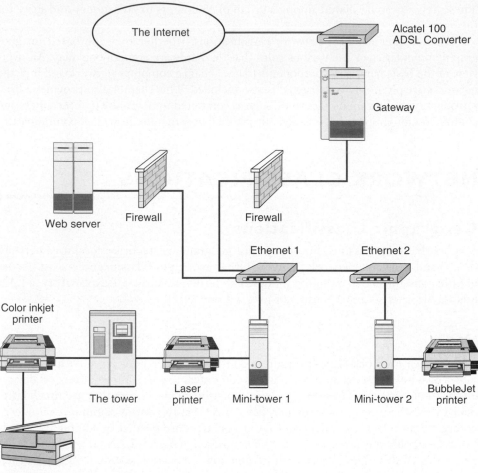

Figure 3-3 Typical office local area network.

what role the computers play in the network's operation and which computer controls the network operation.

Peer-to-Peer Network

In a **peer-to-peer network** (Figure 3-5), each computer on the network is considered equal; no computer has ultimate control over another. Each computer controls its own information and operation and can function either as a client or as a server depending on the needs of the other computers on the network. The peer-to-peer network is the most popular small office or home network configuration because it is the least expensive and most simple to set up. But a peer-to-peer network has a limited scope because the maximum number of peers that should be connected is 10. More than 10 causes

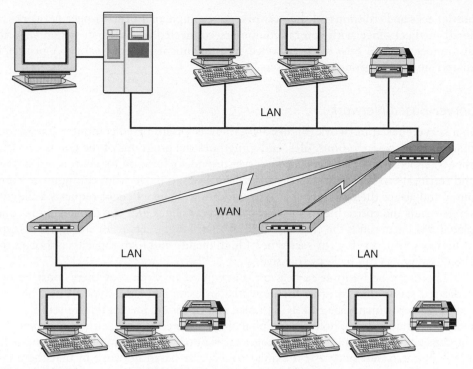

Figure 3-4 Wide area network (WAN) connecting several local area networks (LANs).

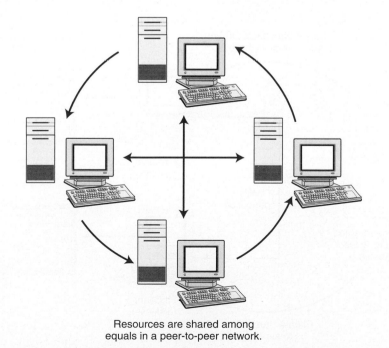

Resources are shared among
equals in a peer-to-peer network.

Figure 3-5 Peer-to-peer network.

bottlenecks and collisions on the network. An example of a peer-to-peer network is a small medical office with several computers connected to check in patients, verify insurance, produce bills for the service, and document patient history. A printer is shared among the group of computers.

Server-Based Network

In a **server-based network** (Figure 3-6), there is a centralized computer (the server) that controls the operations, files, and sometimes the programs of the computers (the clients) attached to the network. The server provides a location for centralized storage and retrieval on the network. This allows the users to move from computer to computer and access their files from a central location. When a client requests a file, the server sends the entire file to the client for processing. Once the processing is completed, the client sends the entire changed file back to the server for storage. This type of network requires that the server be of high quality and high capacity, although the client computers can be less expensive.

There can be multiple servers on this type of network, but there must be one dedicated server that controls the network. An example of this type of network is a radiology department using a PACS to read and distribute images throughout the hospital. Computers throughout the hospital are connected to the centralized server that contains all of the images, and the images are sent out to the computers as requested.

A **client-based network** is similar to a server-based network in that there is a centralized computer that controls the operations of the network; however, rather

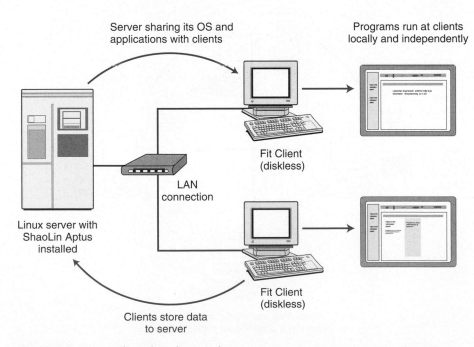

Figure 3-6 Server/client-based network.

than sending the entire original resource to the client for processing, the server processes the resource as requested by the client and returns only the results back to the client. This smaller exchange of information cuts down the load on the network and allows more room for other requests.

TYPICAL COMPONENTS OF A NETWORK

Computers

Typically there are three types of computers found on a network: servers, thin-client, and thick-client (Figure 3-7). Each of the three has a specific purpose on the network.

A **server** is a computer that manages resources for other computers, servers, and networked devices. It may also house applications, provide storage for files, or manage various other networked tasks. A server is most often dedicated to one task for the network and is usually the most robust computer on the network. There may be one server that provides storage for files, one that manages the print functions, and another that provides Internet access for the network.

A **thin-client** is a device that is found on a network that requests services and resources from a server. The thin-client may be another computer, a printer, or any other networkable device that needs a server to complete its tasks. Almost any personal computer (PC) can be a client, as long as it can be attached to the network.

A **thick-client** is a computer that can work independently of the network and process and manage its own files. The thick-client is networked so that it can share resources such as printing and take advantage of the additional security available on networks through dedicated servers. A thick-client is generally a high-end computer that does high-level processing for specific purposes. In health care, specialty application workstations (thick-client) are most often found in cross-sectional imaging modalities for which three-dimensional imaging is used to aid diagnosis. The cross-sectional images are fed into the workstation's application, and the application transforms the slices into a 3D image that can be evaluated.

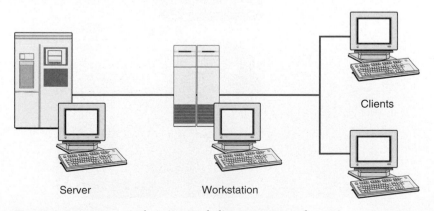

Figure 3-7 A server, workstation, and client on a network.

Network Connectivity

Communication Medium

Once it has been determined what files and resources are to be shared and the pieces of equipment are in place, they are connected via some sort of communication medium. The physical connection between the devices is one of four types: coaxial cable, twisted-pair wire, fiberoptic cable, or electromagnetic waves. Several factors determine which type of communication medium is most appropriate.

Coaxial cable (Figure 3-8) is similar to the wiring used for the cable television that is run into a house. This type of cable consists of a center conducting wire surrounded by insulation and then a grounded shield of braided wire. The shield minimizes electrical and radio frequency interference. Coaxial cable is the sturdiest wire used and is often found in the network infrastructure throughout a building. It is often connected to another type of communication medium before it meets the device interface.

Twisted-pair wire (Figure 3-9) is similar to telephone wire, but whereas telephone wire has only four wires, twisted-pair wire usually consists of four twisted pairs of copper wire that are insulated and bundled together with an RJ-45 termination. Twisted-pair wire comes in various levels of quality and capacity. The minimum recommended standard is Cat 5 (category 5) cable. It is the most commonly used connection medium in LANs.

Fiberoptic cable (Figure 3-10) uses glass threads to transmit data on the network. It consists of a fiberoptic core that is surrounded by a plastic protective covering. It is

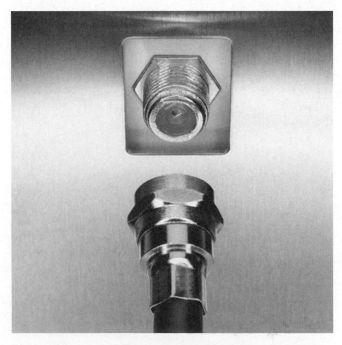

Figure 3-8 Coaxial cable network connection.

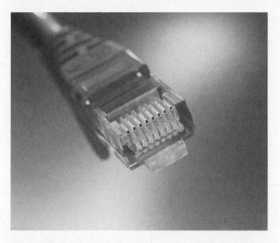

Figure 3-9 RJ-45 jack connected with twisted-pair Ethernet wire.

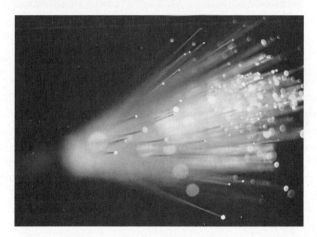

Figure 3-10 The glow from glass fibers in a fiberoptic cable.

much faster than its metal counterparts, but it is more expensive and much more fragile. Fiberoptic cabling can easily be damaged by kinking and twisting the cable. It is most often used in the infrastructure of the network, in network closets, and in large archive/computer rooms.

Wireless connections (Figure 3-11) are becoming more commonplace as technology continues to improve. The connection is made by using either infrared or radio frequencies as its means of communication. There is no physical cabling needed, but each device must contain the appropriate wireless transmitter/receiver. The biggest advantage of wireless connections is mobility and convenience, but it has a limited range. When using wireless access points as the means of connection, the thickness and composition of the wall and the distance from the source must be taken into account.

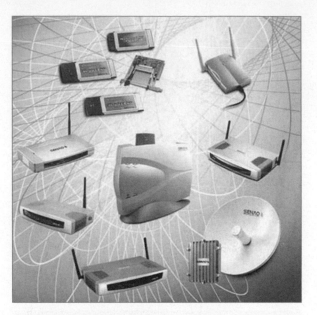

Figure 3-11 Wireless routers.

Network Interface Card

The **network interface card (NIC)** (Figure 3-12) provides the interface between the computer and the network medium; it provides the physical connection between the network and computer. NIC works with networking software to establish and manage the data, to chop up the data into packets, and to handle addressing issues. Most NICs plug directly into the motherboard as an expansion card, but they can also come as small adapter cards that insert into a slot on the side of the portable computer (Figure 3-13).

Network Hub

A **network hub** is the simplest device that can be used to connect several pieces of equipment together for network communication purposes. It has several wiring ports available on it to receive and transmit data to the various connected pieces of equipment.

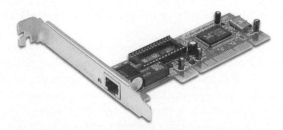

Figure 3-12 Network interface card (NIC).

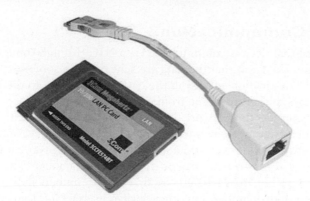

Figure 3-13 External NIC for a laptop computer.

When the hub receives data from a device, it generally sends those data to all devices connected to it. The hub does not know what the data are, nor to which device they should go, so it simply forwards the bits. Hubs are commonly used in small office and home applications.

Network Switch

A **network switch** is similar to a hub, but it sends data only to those devices to which the data are directed. It will read the destination address from the data and select a direct path to the intended target. This reduces the network traffic, speeds up the overall network connection, and makes the network more efficient. In general, switches are not commonly used in small office or home applications because there is not enough traffic to warrant the equipment.

Network Bridge

A **network bridge** is sometimes created so that larger networks can be segmented or broken up into smaller networks to reduce traffic within that network. These segments can then be connected with a bridge. The bridge is a physical (wired) connection from one network segment to another. It can recognize in which segment a particular destination address resides and send data to it. The bridge can also bring two or more networks together that speak the same language (i.e., use the same protocol).

Network Router

A **network router** is a more sophisticated device. It can read portions of messages and direct them to their intended target, even if the device is on a separate network and uses a different network protocol. It also helps with segmenting the network to allow access only for approved devices within that segment. In large networks there will be multiple routers, switches, and hubs that work in concert to perform the necessary tasks that enable the network to perform up to its potential.

Network Communication

We have learned that devices communicate via a NIC through some sort of communication medium. We know that the data are sent through some sort of box and that the box reads the destination address in the data to send them to the appropriate target. So where does the address come from?

Each computer on the network is assigned a unique address. The address is a combination of a physical address from the computer's hardware and a node address given by the network. One type of addressing is Internet protocol (IP) addressing, which is made up of four octets (groups of 8 bits) of numbers. The numbers range from 0 to 255 (e.g., 144.162.21.107). The first set of numbers indicates the network class, and the rest of the numbers tell other devices its exact location. When a message is sent, the computer's NIC will read the destination address and check to see whether it matches the computer's network address. If it matches, it will receive the message. If it does not match, it just ignores the message.

The data travel along the network using an agreed-on set of rules known as a **network protocol.** Most network protocols send data in packets from one device to another. A packet is a piece of the data with added information, such as the destination address, the source address, the sequence of the packets (e.g., 2 of 12), and whether there were any errors in transmission. The protocol is delivered in layers of communication known as protocol stacks. Each layer of the communication represents a particular aspect of network functionality.

Typically a network communication model is explained using seven layers (OSI Model). We need to understand only the basic principles of network communication, so we will simplify the model and concentrate on the bottom four layers.

- Layer 4: The transport layer makes sure data packets are sequenced correctly and that they do not contain errors. For example, the most common transport-layer protocol, the transmission control protocol (TCP), resides in layer 4 and manages the connection for the purpose of controlling the flow of the data packets.
- Layer 3: The network layer breaks up the data into frames and decides which network path the frame will take to its destination. For example, the IP mentioned above is concerned with sending the message to the correct address.
- Layer 2: The data link layer packages the data so that they can be transmitted over the physical layer. Ethernet is an example protocol that performs at layer 2 and layer 1 levels.
- Layer 1: The physical layer consists of the networking media and the components required to pass on a signal from one end of the network to the other. This is the layer that moves bits from one place to another.

The most important thing to understand is that because of this standardized model, different types of networkable machines can be connected to transmit data to each other. As long as the machines share the same low-level protocols or know how to convert from one into another, the packets can be received and reconstructed.

NETWORK TOPOLOGY

Topology is the physical (geometric) layout of the connected devices on a network. There are four common topology configurations: bus, ring, star, and mesh. Many things should be considered when deciding what type of topology should be used, such as the type of communication media, the network speed, the connecting equipment design, and the number of devices to be connected. Each of these four will be discussed in the following section.

Bus

A **bus** (Figure 3-14) is a network in which all devices are physically attached to and listen for communication on a single wire. In a true bus network there is a single point of failure, the wire. If at some point on the wire there is a break, the entire network is down. (In some circumstances communication can take place between the computers on either side of the break.) This type of topology does not need any switches or hubs because the computers simply broadcast all the information down the single wire, and all computers connected to that single wire receive the information.

Ring

A **ring** (Figure 3-15) is a network in which the devices are connected in a circle. Each device passes its received messages to the next node on the ring (always in the same direction), and the data transmissions move around the circle until they reach the correct receiver. If there is a break at some point in the ring, the entire network comes to a halt.

One type of ring topology is called a token ring. The computers are connected in a circle, and a token is transmitted around the ring. When a computer is ready to send a transmission to another computer, it picks up the empty token as it passes by and fills it with the message. As the token passes the other computers, the destination address is read by each passing computer and is ignored if the address does not belong to that computer. When the addressed computer is found, the data are deposited, and the token is now free again. If another computer wishes to send out information but the token is occupied, it must wait until the token becomes free again before it can transmit.

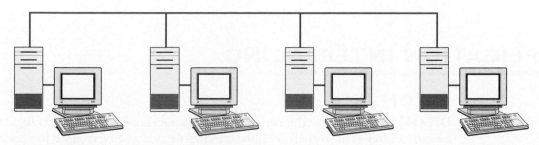

Figure 3-14 Bus network topology.

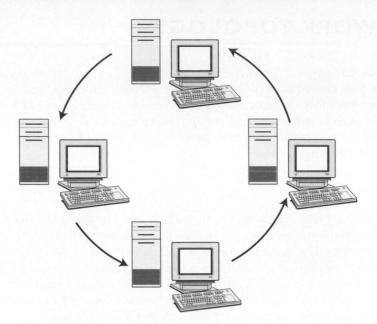

Figure 3-15 Ring network topology.

Star

A **star** (Figure 3-16) is a network that has the devices connected to a central hub or switch. A star topology can be thought of as a bus topology with the bus collapsed into a central box: the hub or switch. The data are sent through the hub out to the destination device. This transmission of data may be through another hub or switch to an adjacent network or directly to the device. This is the most commonly used network topology.

Mesh

A **mesh** (Figure 3-17) is a network that has multiple pathways interconnecting devices and networks. This type of network has redundancy built in with the multiple connections. The Internet is based on this topology, and it is used most often to connect networks to other networks.

APPLICATION INTERFACING

DICOM

DICOM stands for **d**igital **i**maging and **co**mmunications in **m**edicine. DICOM has become an almost universally accepted standard for exchanging medical images among networked medical devices. DICOM is layered on top of TCP/IP, the most common network communication standard used, and it has multiple layers like TCP/IP.

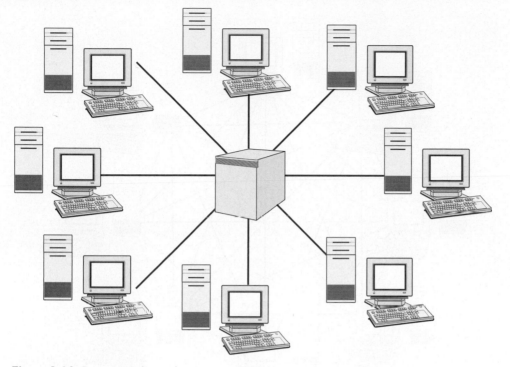

Figure 3-16 Star network topology.

DICOM was developed by the American College of Radiology (ACR) and the National Electrical Manufacturers Association (NEMA). The first version was completed in 1985, addressing only point-to-point connections between devices. At publication of this book, the current version is 3.1. (There are revisions and additions in progress.) Up-to-date information can be found on NEMA's web site at http://medical.nema.org.

DICOM (3.0) was better than its predecessors for several reasons:

- It required a communications protocol that runs on top of TCP/IP (or other standardized protocol stack), permitting the devices to make use of commercial hardware and software.
- It required strict contents of the image "header" and the structure of the pixel data itself for each type of modality, therefore improving interoperability.
- It required a conformance system, so that a user could determine from the vendor's documentation whether the devices would operate together.
- It embraced an open standard of development between the vendors and users to come to consensus on the direction of the standards.

The DICOM standard is made up of 16 different parts ranging from image display to media storage. Not every device conforms to every part of the DICOM, but rather a device will conform to the parts that are necessary to perform the tasks it is assigned according to what is desired by the user. The standard is maintained on a

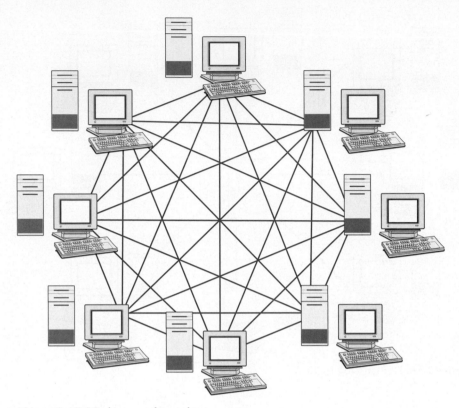

Figure 3-17 Mesh network topology.

continuous basis and is published periodically. Supplements are published with new updates and error corrections, and new parts are being investigated as new functions are developed. Table 3-1 shows the 16 parts and their corresponding titles.

The DICOM standard defines so-called service classes or functions that a device can perform on a defined information object (like a CT image). The allowed service/object pairs (SOPs) for a device are spelled out explicitly in the device's DICOM conformance statement. A device performs either as a service class user (SCU) for a given service and object or as a service class provider (SCP) or as both. The SCU and SCP are commonly referred to as roles. Network communications (i.e., transactions) in DICOM are always between an SCP and an SCU. The most common service classes seen in modalities and PACS are:

- Image storage
- Query/retrieval
- Print
- Modality worklist
- Modality performed procedure
- Storage commitment
- Interchange media storage

TABLE 3-1   THE 16 PARTS OF THE DICOM STANDARD 3.1 (2004)

Part 1   Introduction and overview

Part 2   Conformance

Part 3   Information object definitions

Part 4   Service class specifications

Part 5   Data structures and encoding

Part 6   Data dictionary

Part 7   Message exchange

Part 8   Network communication support for message exchange

Part 9   Media storage and file format for media interchange

Part 10   Media storage application profiles

Part 11   Media formats and physical media for media interchange

Part 12   Grayscale standard display function

Part 13   Security and system management profiles

Part 14   Content mapping resource

Part 15   Explanatory information

Part 16   Web access to DICOM-persistent objects (WADO)

Each of these services defines a specific transaction for the modality and PACS, and because of the standardization provided by DICOM, device interoperability is possible (or at least more likely). The DICOM conformance statement of a device details the various SOPs and possible roles that the modality or workstation can fulfill with those SOPs. For example, if a magnetic resonance imaging (MRI) scanner conformance statement lists the MRI storage SOP class in the SCU role, and the receiving PACS archive lists MRI storage SOP class in the SCP role, the MRI scanner would be able to send images to the archive based on those statements. If either statement does not support the proper SOP class and role, the transfer is not possible. Most modalities manufactured today are DICOM conformant. The vendors will provide conformance statements, and the buyer must closely inspect these statements to ensure that the modalities can communicate with existing image viewing devices.

DICOM also has specifications for uniquely identifying each study, series, and image (instance). DICOM uses unique identifiers (UIDs) to globally identify each image set, so that if the images are sent to multiple systems, the identifying number will remain unique and not get confused with those images on other systems. Each study is identified by a study instance UID, which breaks down into series instance UIDs, and further into instance UIDs. The numbers are created based on a vendor number, serial number of the equipment, date, time, patient or processing number, and then the study, series, or image number. A typical study instance UID may look like this: 1.2.840.8573.4567.1.20051011764589.8765.1.

DICOM also provides a framework for the use of compression technologies on image data. For example, DICOM accommodates joint photographic experts group (JPEG) lossless compression of 2 to 1. This is the most common compression technique used within hospitals because there is no image degradation on viewing after decompression. But when moving images outside of the hospital, it may be necessary to use lossy compression to shrink the file size to suit external networks. Some loss of image detail can occur when higher compression values are used.

When a patient arrives for a procedure, the technologist either has to manually type in the patient's demographics, risking error, or alternatively pull the information directly from the radiology information system (RIS). A modality can pull this information when it supports the service class of modality worklist management, and the RIS can either interface via DICOM or through a gateway that creates an interface with the health level 7 (HL-7) device and the DICOM device.

HL-7

HL-7 is an American National Standards Institute (ANSI)–accredited Standards Developing Organization (SDO).

It is used in most health care applications such as medical devices, imaging, insurance, and pharmacy. The HL-7 standard oversees most clinical and administrative data such as demographics, reports, claims, and orders. As with DICOM, HL-7 is composed of many parts and is used at many levels within various hospital systems. It is the standard generally used in communication between the **hospital information system (HIS)** and the **radiology information system (RIS).** The HIS holds the patient's full medical information, from hospital billing to the inpatient ordering system. The RIS holds all radiology-specific patient data, from the patient scheduling information to the radiologist's dictated and transcribed report. The electronic medical record (EMR) has recently come to the forefront of information technology. The EMR is either a part of the HIS or runs along with it and contains all of the patient's record, including lab results, radiology reports, pathology results, and nurses' and doctors' notes. The EMR interfaces with most of the ancillary service systems to retrieve reports so that they can be viewed in this one common format. PACS have also begun interfacing with EMRs to present images to referring physicians through the same common system.

SUMMARY

- A network is defined as two or more objects sharing resources and information.
- A network can be classified into two major geographic categories: LAN and WAN. There are two typical classifications of networks based on the roles that various components play: peer-to-peer and server/client-based.
- A server is a computer that manages resources for other computers, servers, and networked devices. A client is a device that is found on a network that requests services and resources from a server. A thick-client is a computer that can work independently of the network and can process and manage its own files.

- The physical connection among the devices is one of the following three types: coaxial cable, twisted-pair wire, or fiberoptic cable.
- Information is transmitted via a NIC through a communication medium onto the network and possibly through a hub, switch, bridge, or router.
- The data travel along the network using an agreed-on set of rules known as a protocol.
- Topology is the physical layout of the connected devices on a network. There are four common topologic configurations: bus, ring, star, and mesh.
- DICOM stands for **d**igital **i**maging and **co**mmunications in **m**edicine. It is a universally accepted standard for exchanging medical images among networked medical devices.
- DICOM defines specific information objects and the functions (service classes) that can be performed on them.
- The HL-7 standard oversees most clinical and administrative data such as demographics, reports, claims, and orders.
- The HIS holds the patient's full medical information, from hospital billing to the inpatient ordering system. The RIS holds all radiology-specific patient data, from the patient scheduling information to the radiologist's dictated and transcribed report.

CHAPTER REVIEW QUESTIONS

1. How are networks classified?

2. Define the various network classifications.

3. What are the common network hardware components, and how are they used?

4. What are the different types of network cabling, and what are their advantages and disadvantages?

5. What is the difference between a thin-client and a thick-client?

6. What is the difference between a network hub, switch, bridge, and router?

7. Define network topology, and name the four physical topologies and their characteristics.

8. What is DICOM, and how is it used?

9. What is HL-7, and how is it used?

PART III

Digital Radiographic Image Acquisition and Processing

CHAPTER 4

Cassette-Based Equipment
The Computed Radiography Cassette, Imaging Plate, and Reader

Computed Radiography Equipment

Cassette
Imaging Plate
The Reader

1. Describe the basic construction of a computed radiography cassette.
2. Describe the construction of a computed radiography imaging plate.
3. Identify the various layers of the imaging plate.
4. Describe the purpose of each layer of the imaging plate.
5. Explain the process of photostimulation in the imaging plate.
6. Describe the process of laser beam formation.
7. Explain the process of reading the imaging plate.
8. Compare and contrast conventional radiographic screen and film speed to computed radiography systems.
9. Discuss how an image is erased from the imaging plate.

KEY TERMS

Backing layer
Barcode label
Barium fluorohalide
Cassette
Color layer
Conductive layer
Imaging plate
Laser
Phosphor center

Phosphor layer
Photomultiplier
Photostimulable phosphor
Photostimulable luminescence (PSL)
Protective layer
Raster
Reflective layer
Speed
Support layer

The phrase digital radiographic image acquisition and processing is being used in this book to categorize the different ways of acquiring and processing digital radiographic images. One way to do this is through a cassette-based system commonly known as computed radiography (CR). Another way is through an image detector system that is cassette-less and hard-wired to a computer network and is commonly known as digital radiography (direct or indirect capture; DR). Both systems use computers to analyze and manipulate the image.

The term radiographic refers to general x-ray procedures as distinct from other digital modalities such as computed tomography (CT), magnetic resonance imaging (MRI), and ultrasound (US).

This chapter introduces the basic principles of CR and discusses how CR equipment works. Some similarities between CR and conventional radiography are discussed. A basic understanding of how CR works prepares you to make sound ethical decisions when performing radiographic examinations.

Cassette-based or CR systems differ from conventional radiography in that the cassette is simply a light-proof container that protects an imaging plate from light and handling. The imaging plate takes the place of radiographic film and is capable of storing an image formed by incident x-ray photon excitation of phosphors. The reader releases the stored light and converts it into an electrical signal, which is then digitized.

COMPUTED RADIOGRAPHY EQUIPMENT

Cassette

The CR **cassette** looks like the conventional radiography cassette. It consists of a durable, lightweight plastic material (Figure 4-1). The cassette is backed by a thin sheet of aluminum that absorbs x-rays (Figure 4-2). Instead of intensifying screens inside, there is antistatic material (usually felt) that protects against static electricity buildup, dust collection, and mechanical damage to the plate (Figure 4-3).

Imaging Plate

Construction

In CR, the radiographic image is recorded on a thin sheet of plastic known as the **imaging plate.** The imaging plate consists of several layers (Figure 4-4):

- A **protective layer**. This is a very thin, tough, clear plastic that protects the phosphor layer.
- A **phosphor** or active **layer.** This is a layer of **photostimulable phosphor** that "traps" electrons during exposure. It is usually made of phosphors from the **barium fluorohalide** family (e.g., barium fluorohalide, chlorohalide, or bromohalide crystals). This layer may also contain a dye that differentially absorbs the stimulating laser light to prevent as much spread as possible and functions much the same as dye added to conventional radiographic screens.

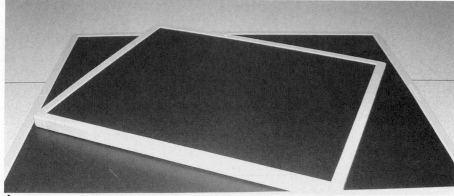

A

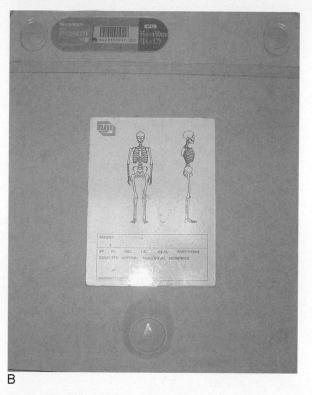

B

Figure 4-1 CR cassette.

- A **reflective layer.** This is a layer that sends light in a forward direction when released in the cassette reader. This layer may be black to reduce the spread of stimulating light and the escape of emitted light. Some detail is lost in this process.
- A **conductive layer.** This is a layer of material that absorbs and reduces static electricity.

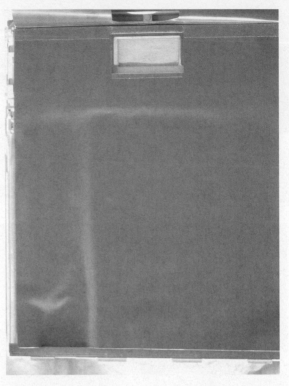

Figure 4-2 Aluminum absorber in cassette.

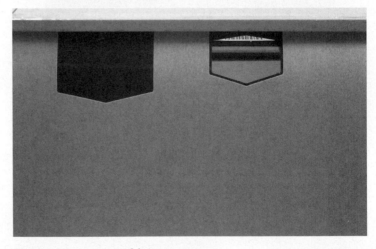

Figure 4-3 Antistatic felt in cassette.

- A **color layer.** Newer plates may contain a color layer, located between the active layer and the support, that absorbs the stimulating light but reflects emitted light.
- A **support layer.** This is a semirigid material that gives the imaging sheet some strength.
- A **backing layer.** This is a soft polymer that protects the back of the cassette.

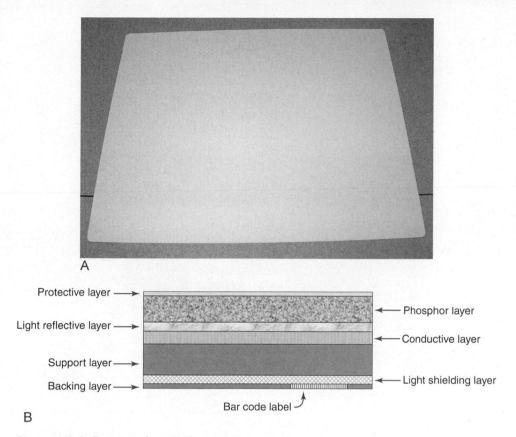

A

Protective layer ⟶ ◀── Phosphor layer

Light reflective layer ⟶ ◀── Conductive layer

Support layer ⟶

Backing layer ⟶ ◀── Light shielding layer

Bar code label ⤴

B

Figure 4-4 A, Imaging plate. **B,** Construction.

The cassette also contains a **barcode label** or barcode sticker on the cassette or on the imaging plate (viewed through a window in the cassette) that allows the technologist to match the image information with the patient-identifying barcode on the examination request (Figure 4-5). For each new examination, the patient-identifying barcode and the barcode label on the cassette must be scanned and connected to the patient position or examination menu. The cassette will also be labeled with green or blue stickers indicating the top and left side of the cassette or with a label on the back of the cassette indicating the top and right sides of the patient (Figure 4-6). These stickers serve to orient the cassette to the top of the patient and the patient's right side so that the image orientation is in line with the computer algorithm. This is discussed more in depth in Chapter 7.

Acquiring and Forming the Image

The patient is x-rayed exactly the same way as in conventional radiography. The patient is positioned using appropriate positioning techniques, and the cassette is placed either on the tabletop or within the table Bucky. The patient is then exposed using the proper combination of kilovoltage peak (kVp), milliamperage seconds (mAs), and distance. The difference lies in how the exposure is recorded. In CR, the remnant beam interacts with electrons in the barium fluorohalide crystals contained within the imaging plate. This interaction stimulates, or gives energy to, electrons in the crystals, allowing them

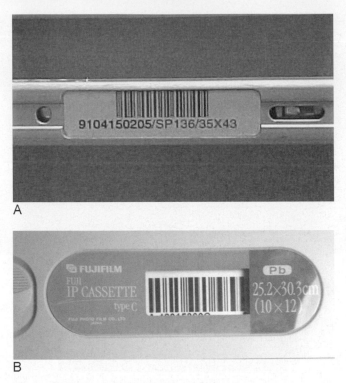

Figure 4-5 Barcode identification labels.

to enter the conductive layer, where they are trapped in an area of the crystal known as the color or **phosphor center.** This trapped signal will remain for hours, even days, although deterioration begins almost immediately. In fact, the trapped signal is never completely lost. That is, a certain amount of an exposure remains trapped so that the imaging plate can never be completely erased. However, the residual trapped electrons are so few in number that they do not interfere with subsequent exposures.

The Reader

With CR systems, no chemical processor or darkroom is necessary. Instead, following exposure, the cassette is fed into a reader (Figure 4-7) that removes the imaging plate and scans it with a laser to release the stored electrons.

The Laser

A **laser,** or light amplification of stimulated emission of radiation, is a device that creates and amplifies a narrow, intense beam of coherent light (Figure 4-8). The atoms or molecules of a crystal such as ruby or garnet or of a gas, liquid, or other substance are excited so that more of them are at high energy levels rather than low energy levels. Surfaces at both ends of the laser container reflect energy back and forth as atoms bombard each other, stimulating the lower energy atoms to emit secondary photons in

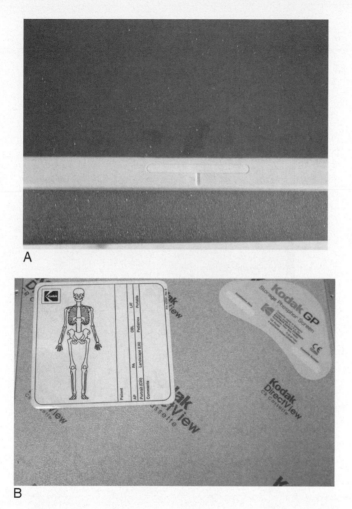

A

B

Figure 4-6 **A,** Fuji cassette orientation stickers. **B,** Carestream (Kodak) orientation label.

the same frequency as the bombarding atoms. When the energy builds sufficiently, the atoms discharge simultaneously as a burst of coherent light; it is coherent because all of the photons are traveling in the same direction at the same frequency. The laser requires a constant power source to prevent output fluctuations. The laser beam passes through beam-shaping optics to an optical mirror that directs the laser beam to the surface of the imaging plate (Figure 4-9).

Using the Laser to Read the Imaging Plate

When the cassette is put into the reader, the imaging plate is extracted and scanned with a helium-neon laser beam or, in more recent systems, solid-state laser diodes. This beam, about 100 μm wide with a wavelength of 633 nm (or 670 to 690 nm for solid state), scans the plate with red light in a **raster** pattern and gives energy to the trapped electrons. The red laser light is emitted at approximately 2 eV, which is necessary to energize the trapped electrons. This extra energy allows the trapped

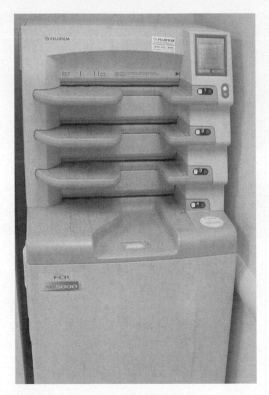

Figure 4-7 Fuji SmartCR CR reader.

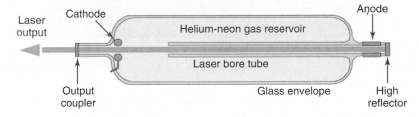

Figure 4-8 Laser construction.

electrons (Figure 4-10) to escape the active layer where they emit visible blue light at an energy of 3eV as they relax into lower energy levels. As the imaging plate moves through the reader, or as the scanning mechanism moves across the imaging plate, the laser scans across the imaging plate multiple times in a process known as translation. Translation can be further divided into **slow scan direction,** which refers to the movement of the imaging plate through the CR reader, and **fast scan direction,** which refers to the movement of the laser across the imaging plate. This scan process produces lines of light intensity information that are detected by a **photomultiplier** that amplifies the light and sends it to a digitizer. The translation speed of the plate must be coordinated with the scan direction of the laser, or the spacing of the scan lines will be affected.

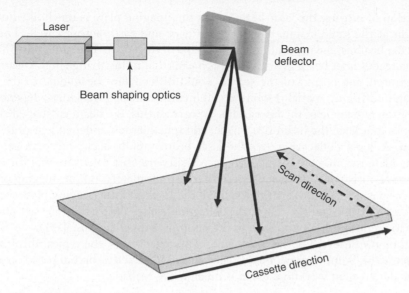

Figure 4-9 CR reader laser optics.

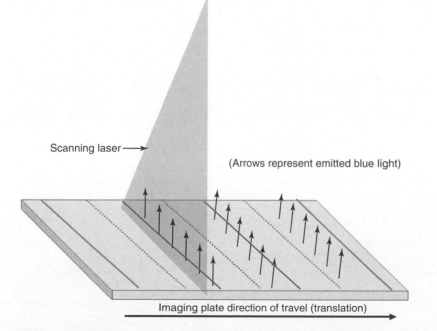

Figure 4-10 The laser scans the imaging plate, releasing stored energy as blue light *(arrows)*.

The action of moving the laser beam across the imaging plate is much like holding a flashlight at the same height and moving it back and forth across a wall. The more angled the beam is, the more elliptical the shape of the beam. The same thing happens with the reader laser beam as it scans. This means that if this change in the beam shape were ignored, the output of the screen would differ from the middle to the edges, resulting in differing spatial resolution and inconsistent output signals, depending on the position and angle of the laser beam. To correct this, the beam is "shaped" by special optics that keep the beam size, shape, and speed largely independent of the beam position. A beam deflector moves the laser beam rapidly back and forth across the imaging plate to stimulate the phosphors. Mirrors are used to ensure that the beam is positioned consistently. Because the type of phosphor material in the imaging plate has an effect on the amount of energy required, the laser and the imaging plate should be designed to work together. The light collection optics direct the released phosphor energy to an optical filter and then to the photomultiplier (Figure 4-11).

Although there will be variances among manufacturers, the typical throughput is 50 cassettes/hr. Some manufacturers claim up to 150 cassettes/hr, but based on average hospital department workflow, 50/hr is much more realistic.

Digitizing the Signal

When we talk about digitizing a signal, such as the light signal from the photomultiplier, we are talking about assigning a numerical value to each light photon. As humans, we experience the world analogically. We see the world as infinitely smooth gradients of shape and colors. *Analog* refers to a device or system that represents changing values as continuously variable physical quantities. A typical analog device is a watch: the hands move continuously around the face and are capable of indicating every possible time of day. In contrast, a digital clock is capable of representing only a finite number of times (e.g., every tenth of a second). In the process of digitizing the light signal, each

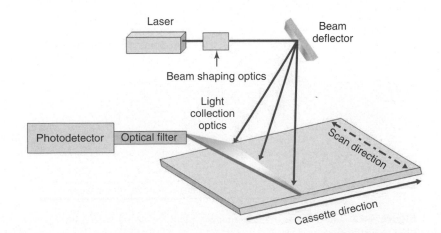

Figure 4-11 Laser optics.

phosphor storage center is scanned, and the electrons are released from their elevated state of excitement causing emission of light that is collected by the light guide. The light is directed to the photomultiplier/charged coupled device that connects the light to an electronic signal. That electronic signal is digitized by an analog to digital converter (ADC). The ADC assigns each picture element or pixel a value that corresponds to a level of brightness. The entire image is divided into a matrix of pixels based on the brightness of each pixel. The typical number of pixels in a matrix ranges from about 512×512 to 1024×1024 for CT but can be as large as 2500×2500 for radiography. As the number of pixels in a matrix increases for the same field of view, the smaller the pixels have to be to fit into that area; the smaller the pixels, the greater the spatial resolution. The image is digitized both by position (spatial location) and by intensity (gray level). Each pixel contains bits of information, and the gray level is determined by how many photons struck the imaging plate in that particular location. The number of bits per pixel is known as bit depth. If a pixel has a bit depth of 8, then the number of gray tones that pixel can produce is 2 to the power of the bit depth, or 2^8, or 256 shades of gray. Some CR systems have bit depths of 10 or 12, resulting in more shades of gray. Each pixel can have a gray level between 2 (2^1) and 4096 (2^{12}). The bit depth will be a factor in determining the quality of the image. A bit value of 21 or one (1) represents a black and white image. The larger the bit depth, the more shades of gray possible. The more shades of gray, the more detail the image can display.

Spatial Resolution

The amount of detail present in any image is known as its *spatial resolution*. Just as the crystal size and thickness of the phosphor layer determine resolution in film/screen radiography, phosphor layer thickness and pixel size determine resolution in CR. The thinner the phosphor layer, the higher the resolution. In film/screen radiography, resolution at its best is limited to approximately 10 line pairs (lp)/mm. In CR, spatial resolution is approximately 2.55 to 5 lp/mm, resulting in less detail. However, because the dynamic range, or the number of recorded densities, is much higher, the loss in spatial resolution is made up for by the increase in contrast resolution. More tissue densities on the digital radiograph are seen, giving the appearance of more detail. For example, an anteroposterior (AP) knee radiograph typically does not show soft tissue structures on the lateral aspects of the distal femur or proximal tibia or fibula. An AP knee digital image shows not only the soft tissue but also the edge of the skin (Figure 4-12). This is a result of the software processing the image data and does not mean there is additional detail. Spatial resolution is discussed in more detail in Chapter 7.

Speed Class

In conventional radiography, **speed** is determined by the size and layers of crystals in the film and screen. In CR, speed is not exactly the same because there is no intensifying screen or film. Digital systems use the terms speed class or speed class of operation. The speed class is a reflection of the amount of light (**photostimulable luminescence or PSL**) emitted by the plate during the reading process and is related to the level of exposure received by the receptor. The level of exposure received by the imaging plate indicates the speed class of operation. For example, Fuji Medical Systems (Tokyo, Japan) reports that a 1-mR exposure at 80 kVp and a source-to-image distance of 72

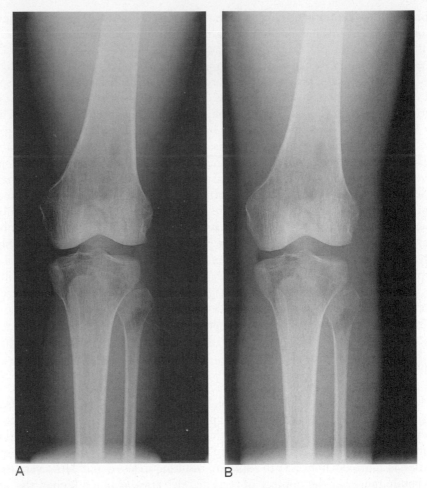

Figure 4-12 A, Film/screen AP knee radiograph. **B,** CR AP knee image. Note the differences in the amount of soft tissue shown in detail.

inches will result in a luminescence value of 200, hence a speed class of 200. Since the speed class is determined by the exposure to the plate, the technologist should use the lowest possible level of exposure factors to produce a quality image. By reducing the exposure to the patient, you will be in essence increasing the speed class. Remember that increasing kV will allow a decrease in mAs needed and will decrease the exposure to the patient. Both the mAs that is necessary and the appropriate kVp value help keep the dose as low as reasonably achievable. More detail about exposure settings for CR systems will be discussed in Chapter 5.

Erasing the Image

The process of reading the image returns most but not all of the electrons to a lower energy state, effectively removing the image from the plate. However, imaging plates are extremely sensitive to background and scatter radiation and should be erased to prevent a buildup of background signal. The plates should be erased at least every 48 hours or when in doubt about the presence of exposure to the plate, under an erase cycle to remove background radiation and scatter. CR readers have an erasure mode that allows the surface of the imaging plate to be scanned without recoding the generated signal. Systems automatically erase the plate by flooding it with light to remove any electrons still trapped after the initial plate reading (Figure 4-13). Cassettes should be erased before using if the last time of erasure is unknown.

Preprocessing, Processing, and Forwarding the Image

Once the imaging plate has been read, the signal is sent to the computer where it is preprocessed. The data then go to a monitor where the technologist can review the image, manipulate it if necessary (postprocessing), and send it to the quality control (QC) station (which may also be the technologist workstation) and ultimately to the picture archiving and communications system (PACS). This process is explored in more detail in Chapter 8.

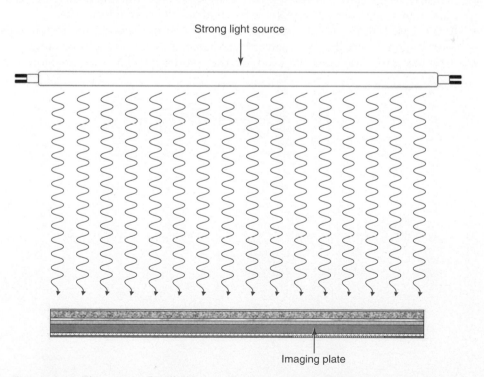

Figure 4-13 Fluorescent floodlight is used to remove any remaining trapped energy.

SUMMARY

- The cassette-based imaging system has a specially designed cassette made of durable, lightweight plastic.
- The imaging plate is multilayered with protective, phosphor, reflective, conductive, color, support, and backing layers.
- Barcodes are used to identify the cassette or imaging plate and examination request to link the imaging plate with the patient examination.
- Barium fluorohalide crystals in the imaging plate release light energy, which is then stored in the conductive layer.
- The imaging plate reader uses a laser to scan the imaging plate, releasing the energy stored in the conductive layer as blue light.
- A photomultiplier amplifies the light and sends it to a signal digitizer.
- The digitizer assigns a numerical value to each pixel in a matrix according to the brightness of the light and its position.
- Spatial resolution of the digital image is determined by the thickness of the phosphor layer and the number of pixels, which also affects resolution of the pixels and the sampling frequency. Cassette-based spatial resolution is approximately 2.55 to 5 lp/mm (lower than conventional radiography's 10 lp/mm).
- Because so many more densities are recorded in CR (wide dynamic range), images have increased contrast resolution but not increased spatial resolution.
- Because *energy* stored in the imaging plate dissipates over time, imaging plates should be read as quickly as possible to avoid losing image information.
- Images are sent to the QC station (which may be the same as the technologist workstation) where they are analyzed and sent to PACS for long-term storage.
- Imaging plates are erased by exposing them to bright light such as fluorescent light.

CHAPTER REVIEW QUESTIONS

1. What are the parts of the digital imaging cassette, and what purpose do they serve?

2. How is the imaging plate constructed?

3. What are the different layers in the imaging plate, and what does each of the layers do?

4. What is photostimulation, and what is its purpose in the imaging plate?

5. How is the imaging plate read?

6. How is the imaging plate erased?

CHAPTER 5

Cassette-Based Image Acquisition

OBJECTIVES

1. Discuss the importance of matching the body part being examined to the examination menu.
2. Discuss the selection of technical factors for brightness, contrast, and penetration.
3. Relate imaging plate size selection to radiographic examinations.
4. Discuss the importance of preprocessing collimation.
5. Discuss the importance of patient side markers.
6. Compare exposure indicators for the major computed radiography manufacturers and vendors.

KEY TERMS

Artifacts
Automatic data recognition
Collimation
Exposure index (EI)
Exposure indicator number
Fixed mode
Focused grid
Grid frequency
Grid ratio
Histogram

Kilovoltage peak (kVp)
Logarithm of the median exposure (lgM)
Milliamperage seconds (mAs)
Moiré
Multiple manual selection mode
Quantum mottle
Quantum noise
S, sensitivity number
Semiautomatic mode
Shuttering

COMPUTED RADIOGRAPHY IMAGE ACQUISITION

This chapter introduces you to the process of acquiring an image using computed radiography (CR). Key topics include selection of appropriate technical factors and equipment selection, exposure indicators, image data recognition, and artifacts.

EXPOSURE

Part Selection

Prior to positioning the patient and exposing the imaging plate, you must select the examination or body part from the menu choices on your workstation. For example, if you are performing a skull examination, select "skull" from the workstation menu (Figure 5-1). Selecting the proper body part and position is important for the proper conversion to take place. Image recognition is accomplished through complex mathematical computer algorithms, and if the improper part and/or position is selected, the image will not display properly. For example, if a knee examination is to be performed and the examination selected is for skull, the computer will interpret the exposure for the skull, resulting in improper brightness and contrast (Figure 5-2). It is not acceptable

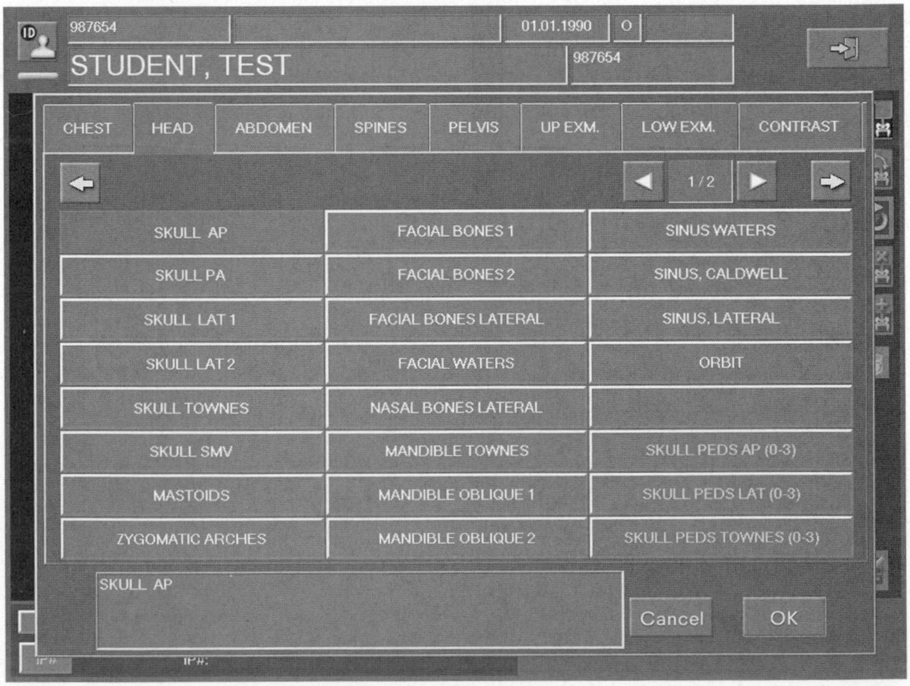

Figure 5-1 Workstation menu skull selection.

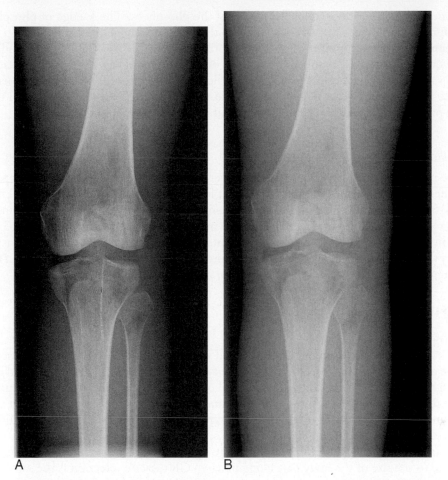

A   B

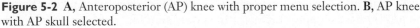

Figure 5-2 A, Anteroposterior (AP) knee with proper menu selection. **B,** AP knee with AP skull selected.

to select a body part or position different from that being performed simply because it looks better. If the proper examination/part selection results in a suboptimal image, then service personnel should be notified of the problem to correct it as soon as possible. Improper menu selections may lead to overexposure of the patient and/or repeats.

Technical Factors

Kilovoltage Peak Selection

Kilovoltage peak (kVp), milliamperage seconds (mAs), and distance are chosen in exactly the same manner as for conventional film/screen radiography. kVp must be chosen for penetration and the type and amount of contrast desired. In the early days of CR, kVp minimum values were set at about 70 kVp. This is no longer necessary. kVp values now range from around 45 to 120. It is not recommended that kVp values less than 45 or greater than 120 be used because those values may be inconsistent and produce too little or too much excitation of the phosphors. The k-edge of phosphor imaging plates ranges from 30 to 50 keV so that exposure ranges of 60 to 110 kVp are optimum. However, exposures outside that range are widely used and will depend on the quality desired. Remember, the process of attenuation of the x-ray beam is exactly the same as in conventional film/screen radiography. It takes the same kVp to penetrate the abdomen with CR systems as it did with a film/screen system. It is vital that the proper balance between patient dose and image contrast be achieved.

Milliamperage Seconds Selection

The mAs is selected according to the number of photons needed for a particular part. If there are too few photons, no matter what level of kVp is chosen, the result will be a lack of sufficient phosphor stimulation. When insufficient light is produced, the image is grainy, a condition known as **quantum mottle** or **quantum noise** (Figure 5-3). Many technologists will choose to utilize automatic exposure controls (AECs), just as they did with film/screen systems. When converting from film/screen systems to a CR system, it is critical that the AEC be recalibrated.

Equipment Selection

Imaging Plate Selection

Two important factors should be considered when selecting the CR imaging cassette: type and size. Most manufacturers produce two types of imaging plates: standard and high resolution. Cassettes should be marked on the outside to indicate high resolution imaging plates. Typically, high resolution imaging plates are limited to size range and are most often used for extremities, mammography, and other examinations requiring increased spatial resolution.

In conventional film/screen radiography, we are taught to select a cassette appropriate to the size of the body part being imaged. CR cassette selection is the same but even more critical. CR digital images are displayed in a matrix of pixels (Figure 5-4), and the pixel size is an important factor in determining the resolution of the displayed

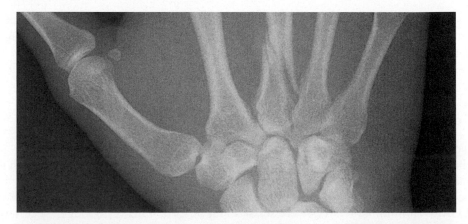

Figure 5-3 Grainy appearance because of insufficient receptor exposure produced in the imaging plate.
(Image courtesy Andrew Woodward, University of North Carolina.)

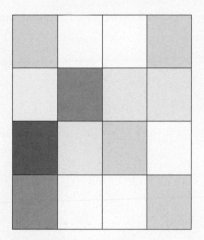

Figure 5-4 Pixel matrix.

image. Some vendors vary the pixel size according to the size of the cassette but some do not. Therefore those systems that vary the pixel size, using the smallest imaging plate possible for each examination, result in the highest spatial resolution.

Grid Selection

Digital images are displayed in tiny rows of picture elements or pixels. Grid lines that are projected onto the imaging plate when using a stationary grid can interfere with the image. This results in a wavy artifact known as a **moiré** pattern that occurs because the grid lines and the scanning laser are parallel (Figure 5-5). The oscillating motion of a moving grid, or Bucky, blurs the grid lines and eliminates the interference. Because of the high sensitivity of CR imaging plates to scatter radiation, the use of a grid is much more critical than in film/screen radiography. Appropriate selection of stationary grids reduces this interference as well. Grid selection factors are frequency, ratio, and focus.

Frequency
Grid frequency refers to the number of grid lines per centimeter or lines per inch. The higher the frequency or the more lines per inch, the finer the grid lines in the image and the less they interfere with the image. Typical grid frequency is between 80 and 152 lines/in. Some manufacturers recommend no fewer than 103 lines/in and strongly suggest grid frequencies greater than 150. In addition, the closer the grid frequency is to the laser scanning frequency, the greater likelihood of frequency harmonics or matching and the more likely the risk of moiré effects.

Ratio
The relationship between the height of the lead strips and the space between the lead strips is known as **grid ratio.** The higher the ratio, the more scatter radiation is absorbed. However, the higher the ratio, the more critical the positioning is, so high grid ratio is not a good choice for mobile radiography. A grid ratio of 6:1 would be proper for mobile radiography, whereas a 12:1 grid ratio would be appropriate for departmental grids that are more stable and less likely to be mispositioned, causing grid cutoff errors.

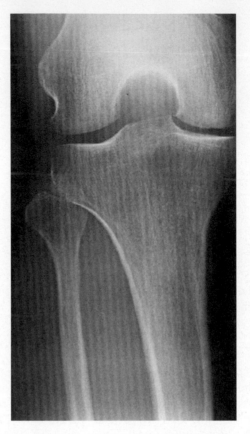

Figure 5-5 Moiré pattern artifact caused by incorrect grid alignment with laser scan direction. *(From Cesar LJ, Schueler BA, Zink FE, et al: Artefacts found in computed radiography, Br J Radiol 74:195–202, 2001.)*

Focus

Most grids chosen by radiography departments are parallel and focused. Parallel grids are less critical to beam centering but should not be used at distances less than 48 inches. **Focused grids** consist of lead strips angled to coincide with the divergence of the x-ray beam and must be used within specific distances using a precisely centered beam.

Collimation

When exposing a patient, the larger the volume of tissue being irradiated and the greater the kVp used, the more likely it is that Compton interactions, or scatter, will be produced. Whereas the use of a grid absorbs the scatter that exits the patient and affects latent image formation, properly used collimation reduces the area of irradiation and the volume of tissue in which scatter can be created. **Collimation** is the reduction of the area of beam that reaches the patient through the use of two pairs of lead shutters encased in a housing attached to the x-ray tube. Collimation results in increased contrast as a result of the reduction of scatter as fog and reduces the amount of grid cleanup necessary for increased resolution. Through postexposure image manipulation known as **shuttering**, a black background can be added around the original collimation edges, virtually eliminating the distracting white or clear areas (Figure 5-6). However, this technique is not a replacement for proper preexposure collimation. It is an image

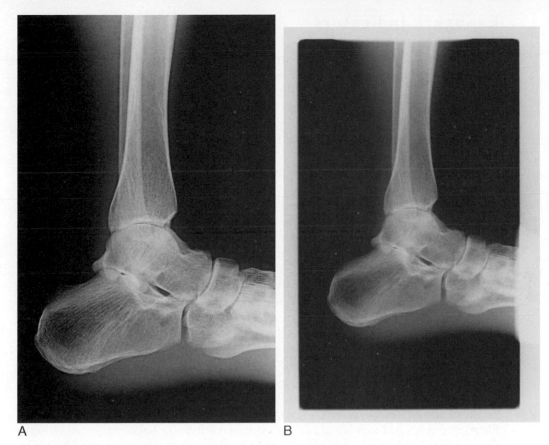

Figure 5-6 A, Lateral ankle without shuttering. **B,** Lateral ankle with shuttering.
(Images courtesy Haley Smallwood.)

aesthetic only and does not change the amount or angles of scatter. There is no substitute for appropriate collimation because collimation reduces patient dose.

Side/Position Markers

If you have used CR image processing equipment, you already know that it is very easy to mark images with left and right side markers or other position or text markers after the exposure has been made. However, we strongly advise that conventional lead markers be used the same way they are used in film/screen systems. Marking the patient examination at the time of exposure not only identifies the patient's side but also identifies the technologist performing the examination. This is also an issue of legality. If the examination is used in a court case, the images that include the technologist's markers allow the possibility of technologist testimony and lend credibility to his or her expertise.

When all of the appropriate technical factors and equipment have been selected, the cassette can be exposed and inserted into the reader. The image will then be displayed. The radiographer must now consider a number of factors: image exposure indicators, image processing modes, and image processing parameters.

Exposure Indicators

The amount of light given off by the imaging plate is a result of the radiation exposure the plate has received. The light is converted into a signal that is used to calculate the **exposure indicator number.** This number varies from one vendor to another (Table 5-1). (The total signal is not a measure of the dose to the patient but indicates how much radiation was absorbed by the plate, which gives only an idea of what the patient received.) The base exposure indicator number for all systems designates the middle of the detector operating range. For the Fuji (Tokyo, Japan), Philips (Eindhoven, The Netherlands), and Konica Minolta (Tokyo, Japan) systems, the exposure indicator is known as the **S** or **sensitivity number.** It is the amount of luminescence emitted at 1 mR at 80 kVp and has a value of 200. The higher the S number with these systems, the lower the exposure. For example, an S number of 400 is half the exposure of an S number of 200, and an S number of 100 is twice the exposure of an S number of 200. The numbers have an inverse relationship to the amount of exposure.

Carestream (Rochester, NY) uses **exposure index (EI)** as the exposure indicator. A 1-mR exposure at 80 kVp combined with aluminum/copper filtration yields an EI number of 2000. An EI number plus 300 (EI + 300) is equal to a doubling of exposure, and an EI number of −300 is equal to halving the exposure. The numbers for the Carestream system have a direct relationship to the amount of exposure, so that each change of 300 results in change in exposure by a factor of 2. This is based on logarithms, but instead of using 0.3 (as is used in conventional radiographic characteristic curves) as a change by a factor of 2, the larger number 300 is used. This is also a direct relationship: the higher the exposure index, the higher the exposure.

The term for exposure indicator in an Agfa (Mortsel, Belgium) system is the **logarithm of the median exposure (lgM).** An exposure of 20 μGy at 75 kVp with copper filtration yields a lgM number of 2.6. Each step of 0.3 above or below 2.6 equals an exposure factor of 2. A lgM of 2.9 equals twice the exposure of 2.6 lgM, and a lgM of 2.3 equals an exposure half that of 2.6. The relationship between exposure and lgM is direct.

A table of recommended exposures to determine the imaging plate sensitivity ("speed class") can be seen in Table 5-2. These ranges depend on proper calibration of equipment and represent the minimum and maximum exposure numbers that correspond with radiation exposure within the diagnostic range. Exposure numbers outside the range indicate overexposure and underexposure. Pediatric examination ranges will vary, as will specific body part indices.

TABLE 5-1   RECOMMENDED EXPOSURE INDICES

	Overexposure	Underexposure	Adult: Nongrid and Grid	Distal Extremities Nongrid
Carestream	>2500	<1600 tabletop; <1800 Bucky	1800–2100	2200–2400
Agfa	>2.9	<2.1	2.1–2.3	2.4–2.6
Fuji/Philips/Konica Minolta	<100	>250 tabletop; >400 Bucky	200–300	75–125

TABLE 5-2	RECEPTOR EXPOSURES FOR DETERMINING IMAGING PLATE SENSITIVITY		
	Carestream	**Agfa**	**Fuji/Philips/Konica Minolta**
Symbol	EI	lgM	S
Exposure factors	1 mR at 80 kVp	20 µGy at 75 kVp	1 mR at 80 kVp
Filtration	Al/Cu	Cu	Al
Sensitivity value	2000	2.6	200
Relative sensitivity	+300 = 2x	+0.3 = 2x	½ S = 2x
x = exposure	−300 = ½ x	−0.3 = ½ x	2x S = ½ x

Image Data Recognition and Preprocessing

The image recognition phase is extremely important in establishing the parameters that determine collimation borders and edges, and histogram formation. A **histogram** is a graphic representation of the numerical tone values of an x-ray exposure. All CR systems have this phase, and each has a specific name for this process. Agfa uses the term "an ROI finder"; Carestream uses the term "segmentation"; and Fuji uses the phrase "exposure data recognition." All systems use a region of interest to define the area where the part to be examined is recognized, and the exposure outside the region of interest is not included in the values of interest used to display the image. Each vendor has a specific tool for different situations such as neck, breasts, pediatrics, and hips in which the anatomy requires some special recognition. The science behind each of these is beyond the scope of this textbook. However, a brief description of the function of four common data recognition modes for Fuji imaging systems will be discussed.

Automatic Data Recognition

With **automatic data recognition,** the image recording range is automatically determined. This mode automatically adjusts reading latitude (L) and sensitivity (S). Collimation is automatically recognized, and a complete histogram analysis occurs. It is critical that good collimation practices are used because overcollimation and undercollimation lead to data recognition errors that affect the histogram. Lead markers must be in the exposure area. Overlapping exposures may have a negative impact on image display, depending on the manufacturer. Current Fuji software is capable of displaying multiple images on one imaging plate, but the trend is to produce one exposure per plate. Each of the exposure regions is processed to identify the shape of the field and the approximate center. Data recognition occurs as the plate is scanned. When the value of the pixels exceeds a preset threshold, those points are interpreted as collimation. Exposure data outside the collimation points are excluded from the histogram analysis.

Semiautomatic Mode

In the **semiautomatic mode,** the latitude value of the histogram is fixed, and only a small reading area is used. There is no collimation detection. The proper kilovolt must be used to maintain subject contrast because the latitude value does not change. This mode is especially useful for examinations of the odontoid, L5/S1 spot film, sinuses, and any other tightly collimated examinations. When using this mode, precautions must be taken to carefully center the part to be examined. This mode is not recommended for high absorption objects such as prostheses. Selection of several different semiautomatic modes may be available where the size of the region of interest is different (5 × 5 cm, 7 × 7 cm, 10 × 10 cm) or with multiple areas of interest where the values of the areas are determined and the resultant maximum value is used such as a PA chest examination.

Multiple Manual Selection Mode

In **multiple manual mode,** the area of interest is selected by the technologist, and the image is derived from the selected areas imaged in semiautomatic mode. Fuji calls this the Semi-X mode, and their user selects from nine different areas on the imaging plate. The same precautions for semiautomatic mode apply to multiple manual mode. The cassette orientation label must be noted with relation to the area of interest. This mode is helpful in cross-table examinations for which the body part may not align with automatically selected imaging plate regions.

Fixed Mode

In **fixed mode,** the user selects the exposure index, or sensitivity number, and the value of the latitude from a menu. There is no histogram analysis and no recognition of imaging plate division. Using fixed mode is like using film/screen: the brightness of the image directly reflects the technique that is used. This mode is useful when imaging cross-table hips, C7-T1 lateral view of the cervical spine, any body part with a lot of metal, and parts that cannot be centered.

ARTIFACTS

As with film/screen, artifacts can degrade images. **Artifacts** are any undesirable densities on the processed image other than those caused by scatter radiation or fog. There are four common types of artifacts (in addition to operator errors that may cause artifacts): imaging plate artifacts, plate reader artifacts, image processing artifacts, and printer artifacts.

IMAGING PLATE ARTIFACTS

As the imaging plate ages, it becomes prone to cracks from the action of removing and replacing the imaging plate within the reader. Cracks in the imaging plate appear as areas of lucency on the image (Figure 5-7). The imaging plate must be replaced when

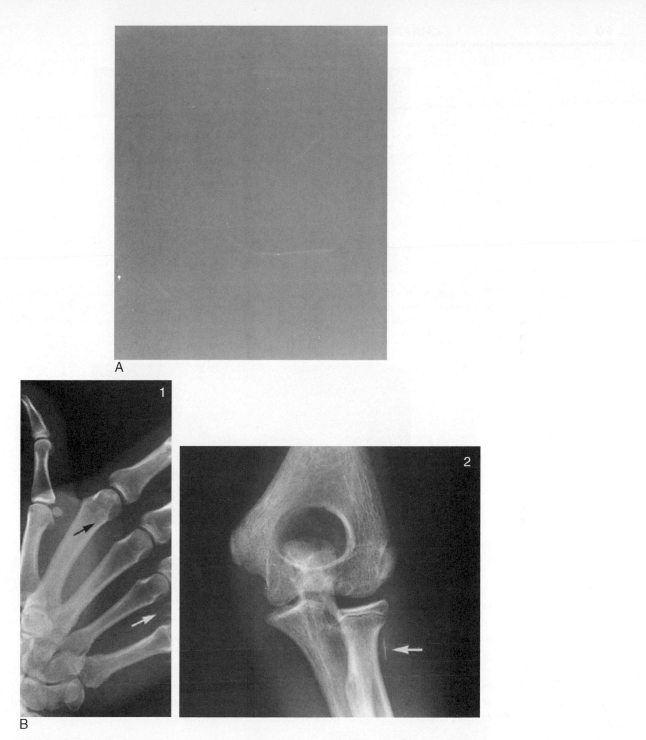

Figure 5-7 A, Cracks in the imaging plate which produce areas of radiolucency. **B,** Imaging plate (IP) artifact. (1) Thumb radiograph showing cracks (white arrow) that usually first become visible on the IP edges. As deterioration progresses, cracks appear closer to the clinically used areas of the IP (black arrow). (2) In some instances, early cracking along the edge of the IP does not occur. This crack appears as a lucency near the radius, which could be confused with a foreign body. (**A,** *Image courtesy Carestream.* **B,** *From Cesar LJ, Schueler BA, Zink FE, et al: Artefacts found in computed radiography,* Br J Radiol *74:195–202, 2001.)*

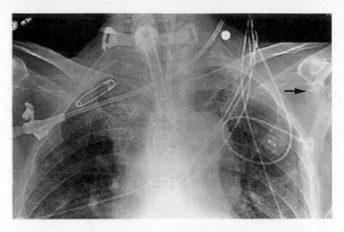

Figure 5-8 Residue from adhesive tape used to attach lead markers to the outside of the cassette has caused artifacts *(arrow)* when the tape came in contact with the imaging plate.
(From Cesar LJ, Schueler BA, Zink FE, et al: Artefacts found in computed radiography, Br J Radiol *74:195–202, 2001.)*

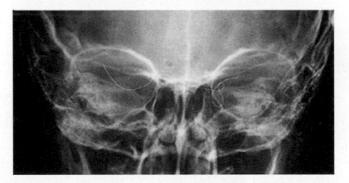

Figure 5-9 Static caused a hair to cling to the IP on this skull image.
(From Cesar LJ, Schueler BA, Zink FE, et al: Artefacts found in computed radiography, Br J Radiol *74:195-202, 2001.)*

cracks occur in clinically useful areas. Adhesive tape used to secure lead markers to the cassette can leave residue on the imaging plate (Figure 5-8). If static exists because of low humidity, hair can cling to the imaging plate, creating another type of image plate artifact (Figure 5-9).

Backscatter created by x-ray photons transmitted through the back of the cassette can cause dark line artifacts (Figure 5-10). Areas of the lead coating on the cassette that are worn or cracked allow scatter to image these weak areas. Proper collimation and regular cassette inspection help to eliminate this problem.

Plate Reader Artifacts

The intermittent appearance of extraneous line patterns can be caused by problems in the plate reader's electronics (Figure 5-11). Reader electronics may have to be replaced to remedy this problem.

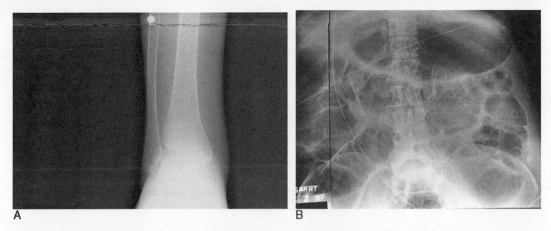

A   B

Figure 5-10 Backscatter causing dark line artifacts on AP ankle (**A**) and imaging plate artifact (**B**). The dark line along the lateral portion of this upper abdomen is caused by backscatter transmitted through the back of the cassette. The line corresponds to the cassette hinge where the lead coating was weakened or cracked. Artifact remedy: to reduce backscatter, the radiographer should collimate when possible. Since backscatter cannot be eliminated in every case, knowledge of the radiographic appearance of cassette backs is useful.
(From Cesar LJ, Schueler BA, Zink FE, et al: Artefacts found in computed radiography, Br J Radiol *74:195–202, 2001.)*

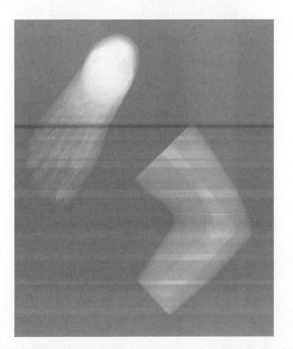

Figure 5-11 Extraneous line patterns caused by noise in the plate reader electronics.
(Image courtesy Carestream.)

Horizontal white lines may be caused by dirt on the light guide in the plate reader. Service personnel will need to clean the light guide.

If the plate reader loads multiple imaging plates in a single cassette, only one of the plates will usually be extracted, leaving the other to be exposed multiple times. The result is similar to a conventional film/screen double-exposed cassette (Figure 5-12).

Incorrect erasure settings result in a residual image left in the imaging plate before the next exposure. The results will vary depending on how much residual image is left and where it is located.

Orientation of a grid so that the grid lines are parallel to the plate reader's laser scan lines results in the moiré pattern error. Grids should be high frequency, and the grid lines should run perpendicular to the plate reader's laser scan lines (Figure 5-13).

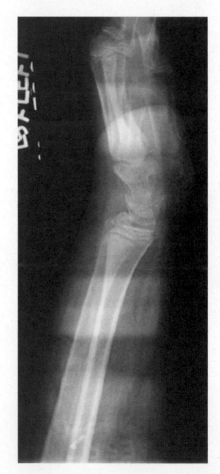

Figure 5-12 This artifact occurred because the plate reader loaded two imaging plates (IPs) in a single cassette. After an exposure, the bottom IP was extracted, read, and replaced as usual, leaving the top IP to be exposed numerous times. Artifact remedy: double-loaded cassettes will be discovered during routine IP cleaning. If a cassette containing two IPs is discovered, the IPs should be erased before being put back into use.

(From Cesar LJ, Schueler BA, Zink FE, et al: Artefacts found in computed radiography, Br J Radiol 74:195–202, 2001.)

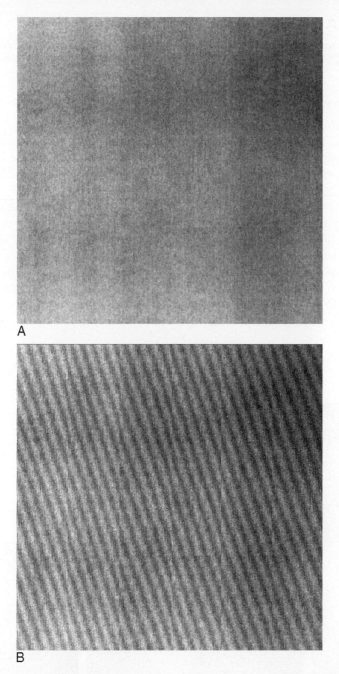

Figure 5-13 **A,** An exposure of a correctly oriented grid with the grid lines perpendicular to the plate reader's scan lines. **B,** A moiré pattern caused by an incorrectly oriented grid, with the grid lines parallel to the plate reader's scan lines.
(Images courtesy Carestream.)

Printer Artifacts

Fine white lines may appear on the image because of debris on the mirror in the laser printer. Service personnel will need to clean the printer.

Operator Errors

Insufficient collimation results in unattenuated radiation striking the imaging plate (Figure 5-14). The resulting histogram will be changed so that it is outside the normal exposure indicator range for the body part selected. Using the smallest imaging plate possible and proper collimation, especially on small or thin patients, will eliminate this error.

If the cassette is exposed with the back of a cassette toward the source, the result will be an image with a white grid-type pattern and white areas that correspond to the hinges. Care should be taken to expose only the tube side of the cassette (Figure 5-15).

Underexposure produces quantum mottle, and overexposure affects contrast. The proper selection of technical factors is critical for both patient dose, image quality, and to ensure the appropriate production of light from the imaging plate (Figure 5-16).

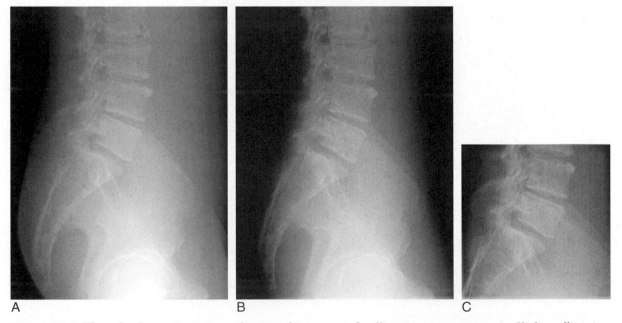

A   B   C

Figure 5-14 Three lumbar spine images showing the impact of collimation on contrast. **A,** Slight collimation. **B,** Increased collimation. **C,** Tight collimation. Note the increase in contrast due to scatter reduction. *(Image courtesy Andrew Woodward, University of North Carolina.)*

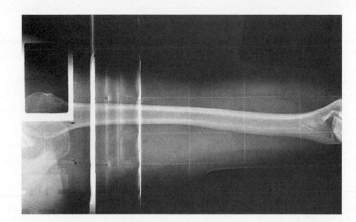

Figure 5-15 This axillary shoulder was exposed through the back of a cassette. Artifact remedy: be sure radiographers are well educated about how to use the entire computed radiography system. *(From Cesar LJ, Schueler BA, Zink FE, et al: Artefacts found in computed radiography,* Br J Radiol *74:195–202, 2001.)*

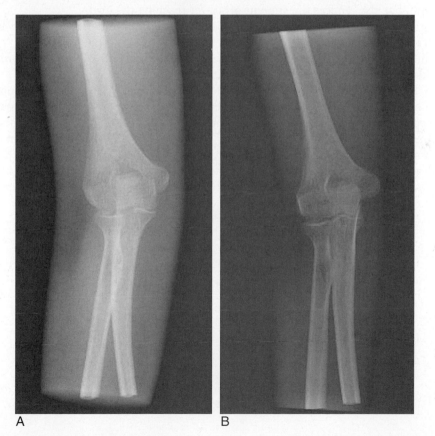

A   B

Figure 5-16 Contrast reduction due to overexposure. The window width and window level settings are identical for these images. **A** had the proper amount of exposure and **B** was grossly overexposed and could not be manipulated to the point where the full range of soft tissue could be seen. *(Image courtesy Andrew Woodward, University of North Carolina.)*

SUMMARY

- Menu choices are critical to proper image acquisition. The menu choice must match the part being examined.
- kVp should be selected for the type and amount of contrast desired. Beam attenuation is the same in DR as it is in film/screen radiography.
- Sufficient photons are necessary to form any x-ray image. Insufficient photons result in quantum noise or mottle. Care must be taken not to overuse mAs to avoid quantum mottle.
- Depending on the vendor, selection of the imaging plate may be very important to ensure the proper matrix and spatial resolution.
- Because of the high sensitivity of the CR imaging plate to scatter, the use of a grid is key. Specific guidelines should be followed as to the frequency, ratio, and focus. Care should be taken to avoid the moiré grid error.
- Collimation not only reduces the area irradiated, thereby reducing scatter production, but also reduces the amount of scatter reaching the grid.
- A black background can be added postexposure, eliminating distractive light-transmitting borders.
- Side or position markers should always be used, regardless of the opportunity to add them postexposure.
- S, EI, and lgM are terms used by manufacturers to indicate the amount of exposure. The exposure range numbers represent the maximum to minimum diagnostic exposures. The middle value in that range represents the S, EI, or lgM number.
- Image recognition takes place through computer algorithms that determine collimation borders and edges and histogram formation.
- Four common types of artifacts are plate artifacts, plate reader artifacts, image processing artifacts, and printer artifacts. Operator errors can also create artifacts.

CHAPTER REVIEW QUESTIONS

1. What is meant by matching the body part to be imaged with the examination menu selection?

2. How are technical factors chosen for each examination?

3. Why is the size of the imaging plate important? What determines the choice of imaging plate size?

4. Why is collimation important? How could a lack of collimation affect the image and the examination?

5. Why is it important to properly mark the patient's right or left side with radiographic markers?

6. How do the major equipment manufacturers determine exposure indicators? What are some potential problems of working with more than one system?

CHAPTER 6

Cassetteless Equipment and Image Acquisition

1. Describe the construction of direct and indirect cassetteless systems.
2. Differentiate between direct and indirect image capture.
3. List the steps for x-ray to digital conversion with amorphous silicon detectors.
4. Discuss the function of a charge-coupled device.
5. Compare detector detective quantum efficiency to cassette-based systems.
6. Explain the importance of detector size and orientation.
7. Discuss factors that affect spatial resolution in cassetteless systems.

KEY TERMS

Cesium iodide (CsI) scintillator
Charge-coupled devices (CCDs)
Complementary metal oxide silicon (CMOS)
Detective quantum efficiency (DQE)
Detector size
Direct conversion

Electronic memory artifact
Field effect transistor (FET)
Flat-panel detector
Indirect conversion
Rare-earth scintillator
Thin-film transistor (TFT)

Digital radiography (DR) imaging is another way to record x-ray exposure after it has passed through the patient. Whereas digital radiography includes both computed radiography (CR) and direct or indirect methods of digital image capture, the term DR is used to describe images recorded on an electronically readable device. Unlike CR, DR is hard-wired to the image processing system and is cassetteless. In DR detectors, the materials used for detecting the x-ray signal and the sensors are permanently enclosed inside a rigid protective housing.

FLAT-PANEL DETECTORS

Flat-panel detectors consist of a photoconductor such as amorphous selenium (a-Se), which converts the x-ray photons directly into electrical signals. This category also includes silicon and CCD detectors.

Direct Conversion

In **direct conversion,** x-ray photons are absorbed by the coating material and immediately converted into an electrical signal. The DR plate has a radiation-conversion material or photoconductor, typically made of a-Se. This material absorbs x-rays and converts them to electrons, which are stored in the TFT detectors (Figure 6-1). The **thin-film transistor (TFT)** is an array of small (about 100 to 200 μm) pixels. Each pixel contains a photodiode that absorbs the electrons and generates electrical charges. A **field-effect transistor (FET)** or silicon TFT isolates each pixel element and reacts like a switch to send the electrical charges to the image processor (Figure 6-2). More than 1 million pixels can be read and converted to a composite digital image in less

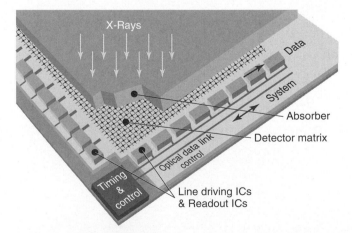

Figure 6-1 Flat-panel detector showing the recording process.

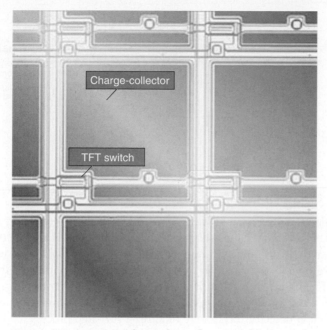

Figure 6-2 Anatomy of an indirect flat-panel detector.

than 1 second. A line of TFT switches, each associated with a storage capacitor, allows the electric charge information to discharge when the switches are closed. The information is discharged onto the data columns and read out with dedicated electronics. Specialized silicon integrated circuits are connected along the edges of the detector matrix. On one side, integrated circuits control the line scanning sequence, and on the other side, low-noise, high-sensitivity amplifiers perform the readout, amplification, and analog-to-digital conversion. High-speed digital electronics are then used to achieve fast image acquisition and processing.

Indirect Conversion

Indirect-conversion detectors are similar to direct detectors in that they use TFT technology. Unlike direct conversion, **indirect conversion** is a two-step process: x-ray photons strike a scintillator that produces light and that light strikes the amorphous silicon allowing the conduction of electrons into the detector. The scintillation layer in the imaging plate is excited by x-ray photons, and the scintillator reacts by producing visible light. This visible light then strikes the amorphous silicon that conducts electrons down into the detector directly below the area where the light struck. A FET or silicon TFT isolates each pixel element and reacts like a switch to send the electrical charges to the image processor. As with direct conversion, more than 1 million pixels can be read and converted to a composite digital image in less than 1 second (Figure 6-3).

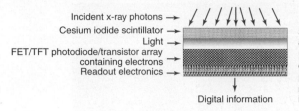

Incident x-ray photons →
Cesium iodide scintillator →
Light →
FET/TFT photodiode/transistor array
containing electrons →
Readout electronics →

Scintillator absorbs x-rays
and converts them to light

FET/TFT array absorbs light and
converts it to electronic charges

Each pixel is read digitally by low
noise electronics and sent to the
image processor

Digital information

Figure 6-3 Thin-film transistor.

Amorphous Silicon Detector

This type of flat-panel sensor uses thin films of silicon integrated with arrays of photodiodes. These photodiodes are coated with a crystalline **cesium iodide (CsI) scintillator** or a **rare-earth scintillator** (terbium-doped gadolinium dioxide sulfide). When these scintillators are struck by x-rays, visible light is emitted proportionate to the incident x-ray energy. The light photons are then converted into an electric charge by the photodiode arrays. Unlike the selenium-based system used for direct conversion, this type of indirect-conversion detector technology requires a two-step process for x-ray detection. The scintillator converts the x-ray beams into visible light, and light is then converted into an electric charge by photodetectors, such as amorphous silicon photodiodes.

CsI Detectors

A newer type of amorphous silicon detector uses a CsI scintillator. The scintillator is made by growing very thin crystalline needles (5μm wide) that work as light-directing tubes, much like fiberoptics (Figure 6-4). This allows greater detection of x-rays, and because there is almost no light spread, there is much greater contrast resolution. These needles absorb the x-ray photons and convert their energy into light, channeling it to the amorphous silicon photodiode array. As the light hits the array, the charge on each of the photodiodes decreases in proportion to the light received. Each photodiode represents a pixel, and the amount of charge that is extracted from the detector is what is used to create the image. The detector exists at a certain state of charge prior to being exposed. Once exposed and the electrons captured, a charge is stored and then read out to create the image. This process is very low-noise and very fast (approximately 30 million pixels/sec).

Charge-Coupled Devices

The oldest indirect-conversion DR system is based on **charge-coupled devices (CCDs).** X-ray photons interact with a scintillation material, such as photostimulable phosphors, or CsI scintillators, and this signal is coupled, or linked, by lenses or fiberoptics that act like cameras. These cameras reduce the size of the projected visible light image and transfer the image to one or more small (2 to 4 cm²) CCDs that convert the light into an electrical charge. This charge is stored in a sequential pattern and released line by line and sent to an analog-digital converter. Even though CCD-based detectors require optical coupling and image size reduction, they are both widely available and relatively low cost (Figure 6-5).

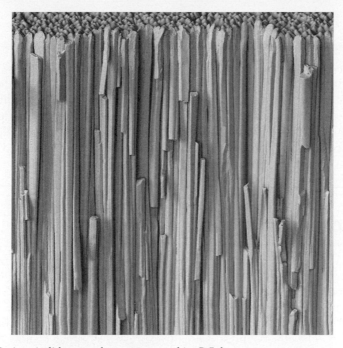

Figure 6-4 Cesium iodide crystal structure used in CsI detectors.
(Photo courtesy Dr. Reiner F. Schulz, SIEMENS Medical Solutions, Vacuum Technology Division.)

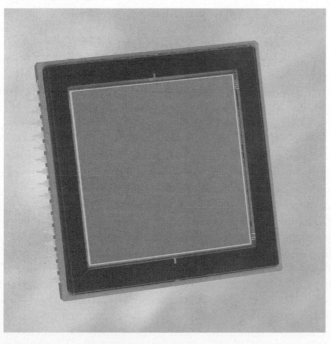

Figure 6-5 Charge-coupled device.

COMPLEMENTARY METAL OXIDE SILICON

Developed by NASA, **complementary metal oxide silicon (CMOS)** systems use specialized pixel sensors that, when struck with x-ray photons, convert the x-rays into light photons and store them in capacitors. Each pixel has its own amplifier, which is switched on and off by circuitry within the pixel, converting the light photons into electrical charges. Voltage from the amplifier is converted by an analog-to-digital converter also located within the pixel. This system is highly efficient and takes up less fill space than CCDs.

DETECTIVE QUANTUM EFFICIENCY

How efficiently a system converts the x-ray input signal into a useful output image is known as **detective quantity efficiency (DQE).** DQE is used to measure the quality of a digital image by looking at the combination of the effects of noise and contrast on the imaging system. Noise, either quantum or electronic, cannot be avoided in digital imaging. The effect of noise is usually expressed as signal-to-noise ratio (SNR). Signal refers to the useful image information and noise refers to information that is not useful to image formation. The more signal you have with less noise, the higher the quality of the image. In other words high SNR, or low system noise, allows the capture of the most useful image information and consequently yields a higher quality image.

Contrast in digital imaging refers to the system's ability to accurately reproduce an object's actual contrast. Digital detectors have a wide dynamic range that allows the capture of a very wide range of signal intensities. In addition, these detectors are able to produce very high contrast resolution, which allows for the display of thousands of shades of gray that can be enhanced with automatic contrast enhancement and window/leveling parameters.

The goal is to achieve high DQE so that there exists the ability to image small, low-contrast objects.

Both indirect and direct DR capture technology has increased DQE over CR. However, DR direct capture technology, because it does not have the light conversion step and consequently no light spread, increases DQE the most. There is no light to blur the recorded signal output; less dose is required than for CR; and higher quality images are produced. Newer CMOS indirect DR capture systems may be equal to direct image acquisition because of the crystal light tubes, which also prevent light spread.

The DQE of detectors changes with kilovoltage peak (kVp), but generally the DQE of selenium- and phosphor-based systems is higher than for CR, CCD, and CMOS systems. CCD in particular has problems with low light capture.

The area of a TFT array is limited because of the structure of the matrix. This also affects the size and number of pixels available. Known as the fill factor, the larger the area of the TFT photodiodes, the more radiation can be detected and the greater amount of signal generated. Consequently, the greater the area of the TFT array, the higher the DQE.

DETECTOR SIZE

Detector size is critical. Detectors must be large enough to cover the entire area to be imaged and small enough to be practical. For chest x-rays, the detector needs to be at least 17 × 17 inches so that both lengthwise and crosswise examinations are possible. Special examinations such as leg length and scoliosis series may require dedicated detectors.

SPATIAL RESOLUTION

Depending on the detector's physical characteristics, spatial resolution can vary a great deal. Noise remains constant in any particular system; however, there comes a point when the most signal that can be captured has been captured and no more is available to increase the SNR. As pixel size decreases, the amount of signal captured decreases so that the finer a matrix is, the lower the SNR will be at each pixel. It should be clear then that there is a balance between pixel size and noise that manufacturers have to work toward in order to achieve the best spatial resolution possible. Spatial resolution of a-Se for direct detectors and CsI, dependent upon detector element size, for indirect detectors is higher than CR detectors but lower than film/screen radiography. Excessive image processing, in an effort to alter image sharpness, can lead to excessive noise. Digital images can be processed to alter apparent image sharpness; however, excessive processing can lead to an increase in perceived noise. The best resolution will be achieved by using the appropriate technical factors and materials.

PIXEL SIZE AND MATRIX SIZE

The amount of resolution in an image is determined by the size of the pixels and the spacing between them, or pixel pitch. More and smaller pixels produce greater spatial resolution. Larger matrices combined with small pixel size will increase resolution, but it may not be practical to use large matrices. The larger the matrix, the larger the size of the image, and the greater the space needed for network transmission and picture archival and communication system (PACS) storage. Typically, 2000 pixels/row are adequate for most diagnostic examinations. Smaller pixel sizes may be necessary for mammographic examinations. Pixel size in TFT displays is related to the design of the capacitance elements and also to the fill factor of these devices.

TECHNICAL FACTOR AND EQUIPMENT SELECTION

Selection of kVp, milliamperage seconds (mAs), distance, collimation, and anatomic markers is the same for cassetteless systems as it is for cassette-based systems. Typically only one exposure is made at a time on the image receptor, but that does not mean that collimation is unnecessary. In fact because of the collimation border/edge detection requirement, collimation may be more critical with PSP-based receptors than it is with TFT devices. When grids are used in any digital imaging system, there is always the possibility that the grid lines will interfere with the pixel rows, resulting in the moiré pattern error. Grid interaction artifacts are not always easy to identify and can decrease image quality, so caution and proper selection of the grid are advised.

POTENTIAL CASSETTELESS IMAGE ACQUISITION ERRORS

Although the conversion of x-rays to a digital signal occurs very quickly, each step of the conversion has the potential of signal loss. While the major cause of noise in any digital system is insufficient radiation striking the receptor, electronic noise can also be a factor. Any noise reduces image quality. The more time allowed for signal conversion, the more precise the pixel values. Incomplete charge transfer will cause inaccuracies in pixel values in subsequent exposures, reducing image quality. Additionally, if exposures are taken in too rapid sequences, there may not be enough time for each previous exposure to transfer the entire signal, resulting in what is known as electronic memory artifact. The detector readout may have built-in safeguards against this, but it would be wise to know whether these protective measures are in place. Not all cassetteless systems are appropriate for high speed, rapid succession imaging such as fluoroscopy. All PSP systems, cassetteless or cassette-based, are susceptible to the same acquisition errors discussed in the previous chapter.

SUMMARY

- There are two types of cassetteless digital imaging systems: direct and indirect.
- Direct sensors absorb x-ray photons and immediately convert them to an electrical signal.
- Indirect conversion detectors use a scintillator that converts x-rays into visible light, which is then converted into an electric charge.
- CCDs act as miniature cameras that convert light into electrical charges.
- Pixel and matrix size are important both in determining the amount of resolution and the size of the image to be stored in the PACS system. In TFT technology, both pixel and matrix size are determined by the amount of area available to "fill" with photons.
- Technical and equipment factors in cassetteless systems are equivalent to cassette-based systems, but both cassetteless and cassette-based technical and equipment factors may be more critical than film/screen in terms of grid use and collimation.
- Incomplete transfer of the signal generated in the cassetteless receptor or the amount of signal retained by the receptor can cause artifacts, especially with short acquisition or rapid succession acquisitions. It should be noted that rapid succession acquisition is difficult to achieve due to newer control mechanisms.

CHAPTER REVIEW QUESTIONS

1. How are indirect cassetteless imaging systems constructed?

2. What are the differences between indirect and direct imaging systems?

3. What are the x-ray to digital conversion steps with amorphous silicon detectors?

4. How does a CCD work?

5. What is detector quantum efficiency? How does the DQE of cassette-based systems compare with detector-based systems?

6. How does the size and orientation of the detector impact digital imaging?

7. What factors affect spatial resolution in cassetteless systems?

CHAPTER 7

Digital Radiographic Image Processing and Manipulation

1. Describe the formation of an image histogram.
2. Discuss automatic rescaling.
3. Compare image latitude in digital imaging with film/screen radiography.
4. State the Nyquist theorem.
5. Describe the effects of improper algorithm application.
6. Explain modulation transfer function.
7. Discuss the purpose and function of image manipulation factors.
8. Describe the major factors in image management.

KEY TERMS

Archive query
Automatic rescaling
Contrast manipulation
Edge enhancement
Exposure latitude
High-pass filtering
Histogram
Image annotation
Image orientation
Image sampling
Image stitching
Level

Look-up table (LUT)
Low-pass filtering
Magnification
Manual send
Modulation transfer function
Nyquist theorem
Patient demographics
Shuttering
Smoothing
Spatial frequency resolution
Window

DIGITAL RADIOGRAPHIC IMAGE PROCESSING AND MANIPULATION

Once x-ray photons have been converted into electrical signals, these signals are available for processing and manipulation. This is true for both cassette-based and cassette-less systems, although a reader is used only for cassette-based systems. Processing parameters and image manipulation controls are also similar for both systems.

Preprocessing takes place in the computer where the image histogram is determined. Postprocessing is done by the technologist through various user functions. Digital preprocessing methods are vendor-specific, so only general information on this topic can be covered here.

COMPUTED RADIOGRAPHY READER FUNCTIONS

The computed radiography (CR) imaging plate records a wide range of x-ray exposures. The entire range of these exposures are placed in a **histogram**. A histogram is a graphical representation of exposure values collected from the imaging plate. If the entire range of exposures were used in image formation, values at the extremely high and low ends of the exposure range would result in a low-density resolution. To avoid this, exposure data recognition (histogram analysis) processes only the optimal density exposure range. The data recognition program searches for anatomy recorded on the imaging plate by finding the collimation edges and then eliminates scatter outside the collimation. Failure of the system to find the collimation edges can result in incorrect data collection, and images may be too bright or dark. Because the information within the collimated area is the signal that will be used for image data, this information is the source of the vendor-specific exposure data indicator.

CR IMAGE SAMPLING

Image sampling techniques will vary from vendor to vendor so as an example of the CR image sampling process, we will use the Fuji Medical Systems terminology in our explanation. For detailed explanations of other vendors' processes, please refer to their equipment manuals.

With **image sampling,** the plate is scanned, and the image's location and its orientation are determined. The size of the signal is then determined, and a value is placed on each pixel. A histogram is generated from the image data, which allows the system to find the useful signal by locating the minimum (S1) and maximum (S2) signal within the anatomical regions of interest on the image. The histogram identifies all densities on the imaging plate in the form of a graph on which the x-axis is the amount of exposure read, and the y-axis is the number of pixels for each exposure. This graphic representation appears as a pattern of peaks and valleys that varies for each body part. Low energy (kilovoltage peak [kVp]) gives a wider histogram; high energy (kVp) gives a narrower histogram. The histogram shows the distribution of pixel values for any given exposure. For example, if pixels have a value of 1, 2, 3, and 4 for a specific exposure, then the histogram shows the frequency (how often they occurred) of each of those values, as well as the actual number of values (how many were recorded). The histogram sets the minimum (S1) and maximum (S2) "useful" pixel values.

Analysis of the histogram is very complex. However, it is important to know that the shape of the histogram is anatomy specific, which is to say that it stays fairly constant for each part exposed. For example, the shape of histogram generated from a chest x-ray on an adult patient will look very different from a knee histogram generated from a pediatric knee examination. This is why it is so important to choose the correct anatomic region on the menu before exposing the patient. The raw data used to form the histogram are compared with a "normal" histogram of the same body part by the computer (Figure 7-1).

The Nyquist Theorem

The **Nyquist theorem** states that when sampling a signal (such as the conversion from an analog to a digital image), the sampling frequency must be greater than twice the bandwidth of the input signal so that the reconstruction of the original image will be nearly perfect. In digital imaging, at least twice the number of pixels needed to form the image must be sampled. If too few pixels are sampled, the result will be a lack of resolution.

The number of conversions that occur in CR—electron to light, light to digital information, digital to analog signal—results in loss of detail. Light photons do not travel in one direction, so some light will be lost during the light-to-digital conversion because light photons spread out. Because there is a small distance between the phosphor plate surface and the photosensitive diode of the photomultiplier, some light will spread out there as well, resulting in loss of information. In addition, even though the imaging plate is able to store electrons for an extended period of time, the longer the electrons are stored, the more energy they lose. When the laser stimulates these electrons, some of the lower energy electrons will escape the active layer, but if enough energy was lost, some lower energy electrons will not be stimulated enough to escape, and information will be lost. All manufacturers suggest that imaging plates be read as soon as possible to avoid this loss.

DIGITAL RADIOGRAPHY IMAGE SAMPLING

Although both indirect and direct radiography lose less signal to light spread, the Nyquist theorem is still applied to ensure that sufficient signal is sampled. Because the sample is preprocessed by the computer immediately, signal loss is minimized but still occurs.

Aliasing

When the spatial frequency is greater than the Nyquist frequency and the sampling occurs less than twice per cycle, information is lost and a fluctuating signal is produced. A wraparound image is produced, which appears as two superimposed images that are slightly out of alignment, resulting in a moiré effect. This can be problematic because the same effect can occur with grid errors. It is important for technologists to look at both (Figure 7-2).

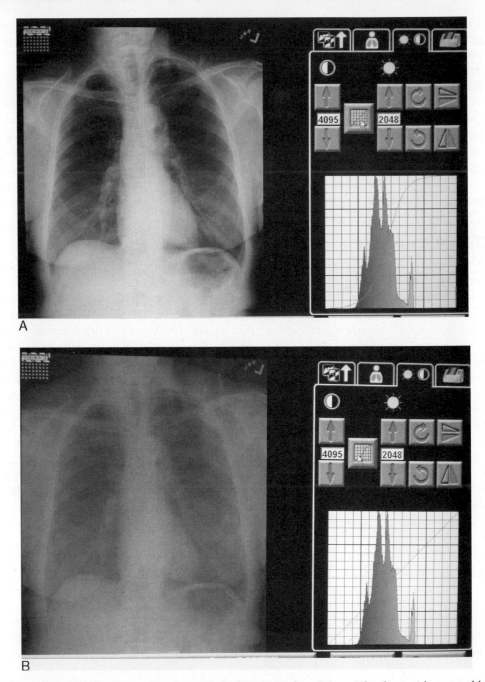

Figure 7-1 Workstation screen showing the histogram for a PA upright chest with acceptable contrast **(A)** and a histogram for the same PA upright chest manipulated to have much lower contrast **(B).** Note that the shapes of the histograms are the same, but the intensity peaks vary slightly. Note the line depicting the "characteristic" curve of the image intensities, which is more vertical in **(A)** and much flatter in **(B).**

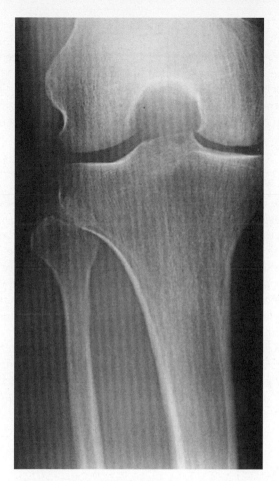

Figure 7-2 Aliasing artifact caused by grid aliasing, also known as the moiré effect. *(From Cesar LJ, Schueler BA, Zink FE, et al.: Artefacts found in computed radiography,* Br J Radiol 74:195–202, 2001.)

Automatic Rescaling

When exposure is greater or less than what is needed to produce an image, automatic rescaling occurs in an effort to display the pixels for the area of interest. **Automatic rescaling** means that images are produced with uniform brightness and contrast, regardless of the amount of exposure. Problems occur with automatic rescaling when too little exposure is used or when too much exposure is used. Quantum mottle or noise is often seen when not enough exposure is used for that particular anatomic body part. Too much exposure will result in a loss of contrast and loss of distinct edges because of detector saturation. Rescaling is no substitute for appropriate technical factors. There is a real danger in relying on the system to "fix" an image through rescaling and so using higher milliamperage seconds (mAs) values than necessary to avoid quantum mottle.

Look-Up Table

A **look-up table (LUT)** is a table of the luminance values derived during image acquisition. The LUT is used as a reference to evaluate the raw information and correct the luminance values. This is a mapping function in which all pixels (each with its own specific gray value) are changed to a new gray value. The resultant image will have the appropriate appearance in brightness (density) and contrast. There is a LUT for every anatomic part. The LUT can be graphed by plotting the original values ranging from 0 to 255 on the horizontal axis and the new values (also ranging from 0 to 255) on the vertical axis. Contrast can be increased or decreased by changing the slope of this graph. The brightness (density) can be increased or decreased by moving the line up or down the y-axis (Figure 7-3).

Exposure Latitude

Exposure latitude refers to the range of exposures that can be used and still result in the capture of a diagnostic quality image. The exposure latitude is greater for digital imaging receptors than that of screen/film exposures. The greater exposure latitude is due to the higher dynamic range of the receptors. Dynamic range refers to the image receptor's ability to respond to the exposure. In CR if the exposure is more than 50% below the ideal exposure, quantum mottle results. If the exposure is more than 200% above the ideal exposure, contrast loss results. The biggest difference between digital and film/screen radiography lies in the ability to manipulate the digitized pixel values, which leads to what seems like greater exposure latitude.

Carestream (Rochester, NY) has added a feature to its CR systems called enhanced visualization image processing (EVP). EVP takes image diagnostic quality to a new level by increasing latitude while still preserving the contrast of image detail. Carestream's EVP process decreases windowing and leveling on workstations and virtually eliminates detail loss in dense tissues (Figure 7-4).

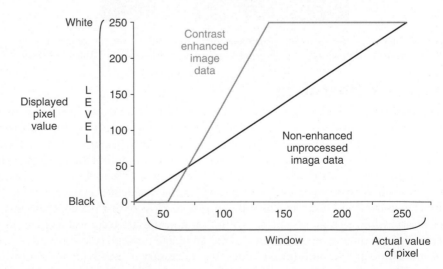

Figure 7-3 Look-up table. Gray-level transformation required for contrast enhancement of images with 256 shades of gray for an 8-bit matrix. The nonenhanced image data are transformed so that data with pixel values less than 50 are displayed as black, and all data with pixel values greater than 150 are displayed as white. All data with pixel values between 50 and 150 are displayed using an intermediate shade of gray.

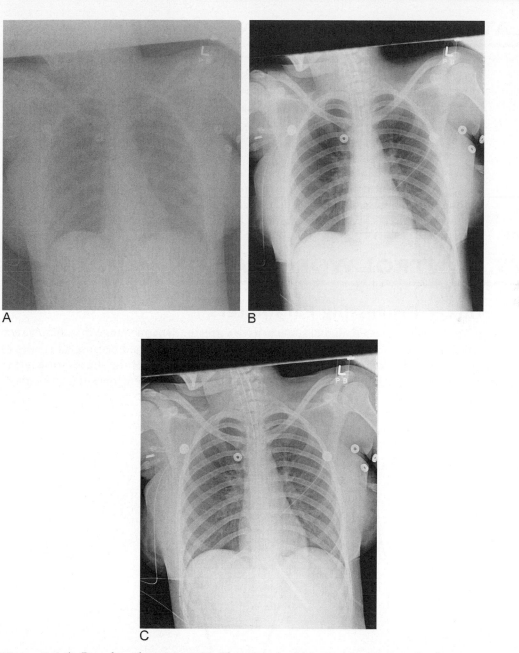

Figure 7-4 A, Raw data chest image. **B,** Chest image with some image processing known as "perceptual tone scale image processing" (ptone). **C,** Final enhanced image using enhanced visualization image processing (EVP).
(Images courtesy Carestream.)

MODULATION TRANSFER FUNCTION

The ability of a system to record available spatial frequencies is known as **modulation transfer function (MTF).** The sum of the components in a recording system cannot be greater than the system as a whole. What this means is that when any component's function is compromised because of some type of interference, the overall quality of the system is affected. MTF is a way to quantify the contribution of each system component to the efficiency of the entire system. MTF is a ratio of the image to the object, so that a perfect system would have an MTF of 1% or 100%. In digital detectors where x-ray photon energy excites a phosphor so that it produces light, there will always be a spreading out of the light that reduces system efficiency. Therefore the more light spread, the less the image looks like the object and the lower the MTF (Figure 7-5).

QUALITY CONTROL WORKSTATION FUNCTIONS

Image Processing Parameters

As previously discussed, digital systems have a greater dynamic range than film/screen imaging. The initial digital image appears linear when graphed because all shades of gray are visible, giving the image a very wide latitude. If all of the shades were left in the image, the contrast would be so low as to make adjacent densities difficult to

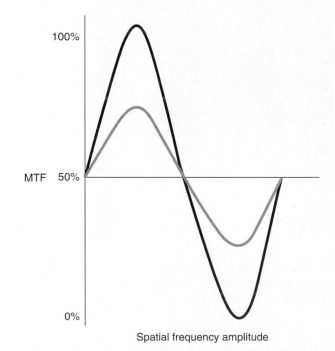

Figure 7-5 MTF comparison. The blue line shows high spatial frequency, which results in an MTF of 100%. The maroon line shows a substantially lower spatial frequency, indicating system inefficiency. The closer the amplitude of the spatial frequency is to becoming a flat line, the lower the MTF.

differentiate. To avoid this, digital systems use various contrast enhancement parameters. Although the parameter names differ by vendor (Agfa [Mortsel, Belgium] uses MUSICA; Fuji [Tokyo, Japan] uses Gradation; and Carestream uses Tonescaling), the purpose and effects are basically the same.

Contrast Manipulation

Contrast manipulation involves converting the digital input data to an image with appropriate brightness and contrast using contrast enhancement parameters. Image contrast is controlled by using a parameter that changes the steepness of the exposure gradient. By using a different parameter, brightness can be varied at the toe and shoulder of the curve to remove the extremely low- and extremely high-density values. Another parameter allows brightness to remain unchanged, whereas contrast is varied. These parameters should be used only to enhance the image. No amount of adjustment can take the place of proper technical factor selection (Figure 7-6).

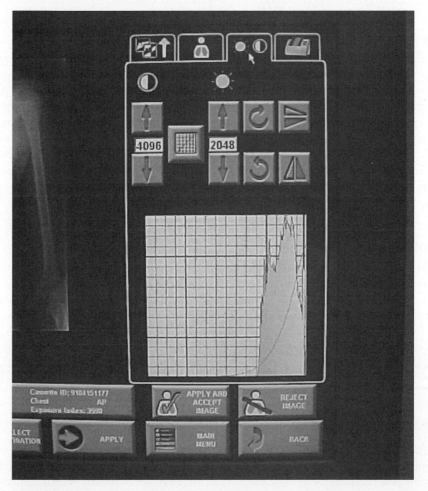

Figure 7-6 Workstation screen showing contrast manipulation choices.

Spatial Frequency Resolution

Detail or sharpness is referred to as spatial frequency resolution. In film/screen radiography, sharpness is controlled by various factors such as focal spot size, screen and/or film speed, and object-image distance (OID). Focal spot and the OID affect image sharpness in both film/screen and DR. The digitized image, however, can be further controlled for sharpness by adjusting processing parameters. You can choose the structure to be enhanced, control the degree of enhancement for each density to reduce image graininess, and adjust how much edge enhancement is applied. Great care must be taken when making adjustments to processing parameters because if the improper algorithms are applied, image formation can be degraded.

Many health care facilities do not want the technologist to manipulate the image much before it goes to the picture archival and communication system (PACS) because their changes reduce the amount of manipulation that the radiologist can do. Once the image is stored in the PACS, all postprocessing results in a loss of information from the original image.

Spatial Frequency Filtering

Edge Enhancement

After the signal is obtained for each pixel, the signals are averaged to shorten processing time and storage. The more pixels involved in the averaging, the smoother the image appears. The signal strength of one pixel is averaged with the strength of adjacent pixels, or neighborhood pixels. **Edge enhancement** occurs when fewer pixels in the neighborhood are included in the signal average. The smaller the neighborhood, the greater the enhancement. When the frequencies of areas of interest are known, those frequencies can be amplified and other frequencies suppressed. This is also known as **high-pass filtering** and increases contrast and edge enhancement. Suppressing frequencies, also known as *masking*, can result in the loss of small details. High-pass filtering is useful for enhancing large structures like organs and soft tissues, but it can be noisy (Figure 7-7).

Smoothing

Another type of spatial frequency filtering is **smoothing.** Also known as **low-pass filtering,** smoothing occurs by averaging each pixel's frequency with surrounding pixel values to remove high-frequency noise. The result is a reduction of noise and contrast. Low-pass filtering is useful for viewing small structures such as fine bone tissues.

BASIC FUNCTIONS OF THE PROCESSING SYSTEM

Image Manipulation

Window and Level

The most common image processing parameters are those for brightness and contrast. **Window level** controls how light or dark the image is, and **window width** controls the ratio of black to white, or contrast. The user can quickly manipulate both by using the

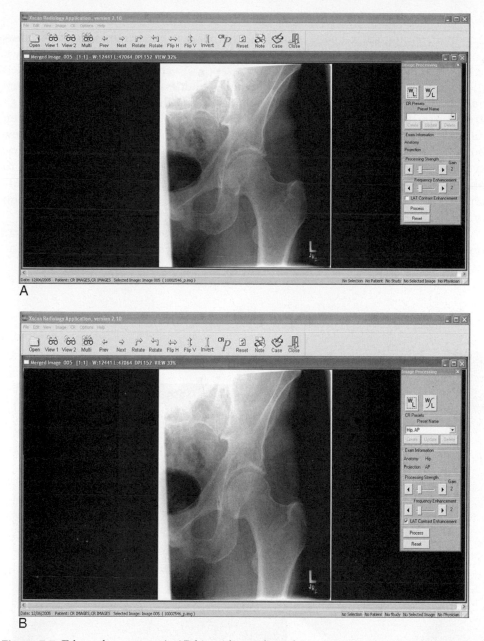

Figure 7-7 Edge enhancement. **A,** AP hip without edge enhancement. **B,** The same AP hip image with edge enhancement.

mouse. Care should be taken, as this may be a permanent change depending on the vendor and could have a negative impact on the image at the radiologist's workstation. Movement of the mouse in one direction (vertical or horizontal) controls brightness, and the other direction controls contrast. To further control brightness and contrast, contrast enhancement parameters are used.

Background Removal or Shuttering

Anytime a radiographic image is viewed, whether it is film/screen or digital, unexposed borders around the collimation edges allow excess light to enter the eye. Known as *veil glare*, this excess light causes oversensitization of a chemical within the eye called rhodopsin that results in temporary white light blindness. Although the eye recovers quickly enough so that the viewer recognizes only that the light is very bright, it is a great distraction that interferes with image reception by the eye. In film/screen radiography, black cardboard glare masks or special automatic collimation view boxes were sometimes used to lessen the effects of veil glare, but no technique has ever been entirely successful or convenient. Automatic **shuttering** is used to blacken out the white collimation borders, effectively eliminating veil glare. Shuttering is a viewing technique only and should never be used to mask poor collimation practices.

Background removal is also beneficial. Removing the white unexposed borders results in an overall smaller number of pixels and reduces the amount of information to be stored (Figure 7-8).

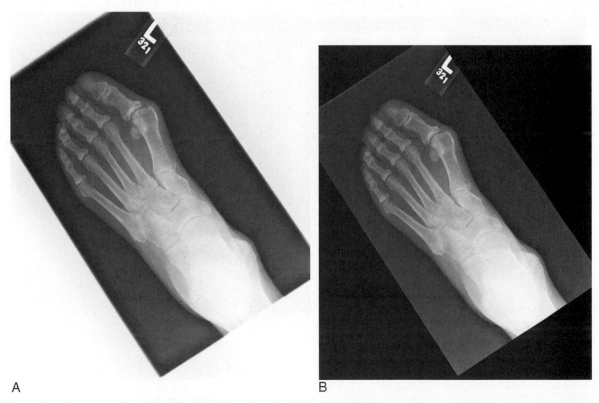

A   B

Figure 7-8 Shuttering. **A,** AP foot with collimation. **B,** AP foot with collimation and black surround or shuttering. *(Images courtesy Carestream.)*

Image Orientation

Image orientation refers to the way anatomy is oriented on the imaging plate. The image reader has to be informed of the location of the patient's head versus feet and right side versus left side. The image reader scans and reads the image from the leading edge of the imaging plate to the opposite end. The image is displayed exactly as it was read unless the reader is informed differently. Vendors mark the cassettes in different ways to help technologists orient the cassette in such a way that the image will be processed to display as expected. Fuji uses a tape-type orientation marker on the top and right side of the cassette. Carestream uses a sticker reminiscent of the film/screen cassette identification blocker. Some examinations, however, require unusual orientation of the cassette. In these cases, the reader must be informed of the orientation of the anatomy with respect to the reader. In DR, for which no cassette is used, the position of the part should correspond with the marked top and sides of the imaging plate.

Image Stitching

When anatomy or area of interest is too large to fit on one cassette, multiple images can be "stitched" together using specialized software programs. This process is called **image stitching.** In some cases special cassette holders are used and positioned vertically, corresponding to foot-to-hip or entire spine studies. Images are processed in computer programs that nearly seamlessly join the anatomy for display as one single image. This technique eliminates the need for large (36-inch) cassettes previously used in film/screen radiography (Figure 7-9).

Image Annotation

Many times, information other than standard identification must be added to the image. In screen/film radiography, time and date stickers, grease pencils, or permanent markers were used to indicate technical factors, time sequences, technologist identification, or position. The **image annotation** function allows selection of preset terms and/or manual text input and can be particularly useful when such additional information is necessary. (Function availability depends on the manufacturer.) The annotations overlay the image as bitmap images. Depending on how each system is set up, annotations may not transfer to PACS. Again, input of annotation for identification of the patient's left or right side should never be used as a substitute for technologist's anatomy markers (Figure 7-10).

Magnification

Two basic types of **magnification** techniques come standard with digital systems. One technique functions as a magnifying glass in the sense that a box placed over a small segment of anatomy on the main image shows a magnified version of the underlying anatomy. Both the size of the magnified area and the amount of magnification can be made larger or smaller. The other technique is a "zoom" technique that allows magnification of the entire image. The image can be enlarged enough so that only parts of it are visible on the screen, but the parts not visible can be reached through mouse navigation (Figure 7-11).

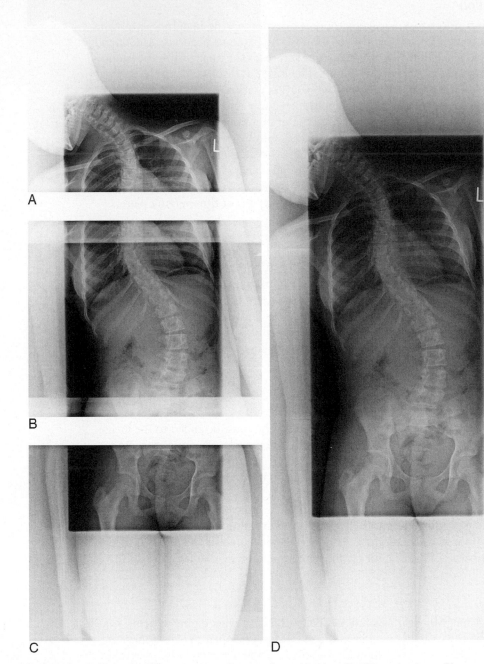

Figure 7-9 Image stitching. **A,** AP projection of upper thoracic spine. **B,** AP projection of lower thoracic and upper lumbar spine. **C,** AP projection of lower lumbar spine. **D,** All three images joined by digital stitching, resulting in AP projection of entire spine for scoliosis.
(Images courtesy Carestream.)

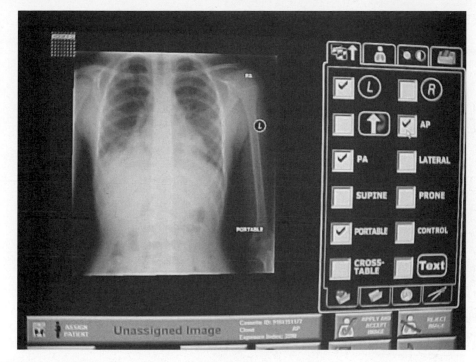

Figure 7-10 CR workstation screen for image annotation. Note that even though both PA and AP choices are checked, only the first (PA) shows on the screen.

IMAGE MANAGEMENT

Patient Demographic Input

Proper identification of the patient is even more critical with digital images than with conventional hard copy film/screen images. Retrieval of digital images can be nearly impossible if not properly and accurately identified. **Patient demographics** include things like patient name, health care facility, patient identification number, date of birth, and examination date. This information should be input or linked via barcode label scans before the start of the examination and before the processing phase. Occasionally errors are made, and demographic information must be altered. If the technologist performing the examination is absolutely positive that the image is of the correct patient, then demographic information can be altered at the processing stage. This function should be tracked and changes linked to the technologist altering the information to ensure accuracy and accountability.

Problems arise if the patient name is entered differently from visit to visit or examination to examination. For example, if the patient's name is Jane A. Doe and is entered that way, that name must be entered that way for every other examination. If entered as Jane Doe, the system will save it as a different patient. Merging these files can be difficult, especially if there are several versions of the name. If a patient gives

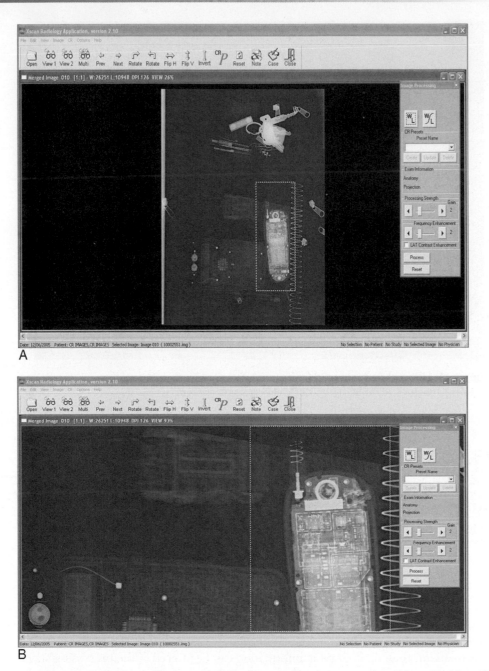

Figure 7-11 Image magnification. **A,** Digital image of various everyday objects. **B,** Magnified view of a cell phone.

a middle name on one visit but has had multiple examinations under his or her first name, retrieval of previous files will be very difficult and in some cases impossible. The right images must be placed in the correct data files just as hard copy films had to be placed in the correct patient folder.

Manual Send

Because the quality control (QC) workstation is networked to the PACS, it also has the capability to send images to local network workstations. The **manual send** function allows the QC technologist to select one or more local computers to receive images.

Archive Query

In the event that the technologist wishes to see historical images, the PACS archive can be queried. **Archive query** is a function that allows retrieval of images from the PACS based on date of examination, patient name or number, examination number, pathologic condition, or anatomic area. For example, the technologist could query or ask the PACS to retrieve all chest x-rays for a particular date or range of dates, or query retrieval of all of a certain patient's images. There are multiple combinations of query fields that can generate reports that include many categories of information or a few very specific categories to be retrieved from storage.

SUMMARY

- Recognition of exposure data involves placing all exposures detected in a histogram. The histogram then undergoes analysis.
- After the plate is scanned and the image location is determined, a value is placed on each pixel, and the histogram is generated displaying the minimum and maximum diagnostic signal.
- Histograms are different for specific anatomic regions and remain fairly constant from patient to patient.
- Automatic rescaling allows pixel display for the area of interest, regardless of the amount of exposure.
- There is no substitute for proper kVp and mAs. Insufficient photons, insufficient penetration, or overpenetration results in a loss of diagnostic information that cannot be manufactured by manipulating the image parameters.
- Exposure latitude is slightly greater with digital imaging than with film/screen imaging because of the wider range of exposures recorded with digital systems.
- Contrast enhancement parameters allow enhancement of the image by controlling the steepness of the exposure gradient, density variance, and contrast amount.
- Spatial frequency resolution is controlled by focal spot, OID, and computer algorithms.
- The Nyquist theorem is applied to digital images to ensure sufficient signal sampling for maximum resolution.

- MTF refers to the contribution of all system components to total resolution. The closer the MTF value is to 1, the better the resolution.

- Edge enhancement is accomplished by limiting the number of pixels in a neighborhood of the matrix. Known area-of-interest frequencies can be amplified or high-pass filtered to increase contrast and edge enhancement.

- Suppressing frequencies of lesser importance, known as *masking*, can cause small detail loss.

- Low-pass filtering or smoothing is the result of pixel averaging to remove high frequency noise. Contrast and noise are decreased, allowing small structures to be seen.

- Window and level parameters control pixel brightness and contrast.

- Shuttering is a process that removes or replaces the background to block distracting light surrounding a digital image. This does not take the place of proper collimation and can be removed to show proper collimation.

- Digital imaging cassettes are marked for orientation to the top and right sides. This ensures that images will be displayed correctly.

- Image stitching is a computer program process that allows multiple images to be joined when the anatomy is too large for one exposure. The result is a nearly seamless single image.

- On digital systems, magnification techniques are available that allow small area enlargement or whole image enlargement.

- Proper patient demographic input is the responsibility of the technologist performing the examination. Any alteration of patient demographics should be avoided unless absolute identification is possible.

- The manual send function allows images to be sent to one or more networked computers.

- Historical study of patient examinations can be accomplished through the archive query function. Querying for retrieval of radiographic studies can be specific to a patient, examination date, or examination type or include a broader search for date ranges, combinations of anatomic areas, and so on.

CHAPTER REVIEW QUESTIONS

1. What is an image histogram?

2. How is the image histogram formed?

3. What is the purpose of automatic rescaling?

4. How does image latitude in digital imaging compare with film/screen radiography?

5. What is the Nyquist theorem? How does it affect digital image processing?

6. What happens if the incorrect algorithm is applied to an examination?

7. What does image manipulation mean? What are the different types of manipulation choices, and what are their functions?

8. What are the major factors in image management?

PART IV

PACS

PACS Fundamentals

1. Define picture archiving and communication system (PACS).
2. Compare and contrast the various types of PACS display workstations.
3. Differentiate among the different types of digital imaging workflow.

4. Define system architecture, and recognize the three major models.
5. Summarize the common functions found on a PACS workstation.
6. Describe the situations and users that may require advanced PACS workstation functions.

Archive
Client/server-based system
Digital imaging and communications in medicine (DICOM)
Display workstation
Distributed or stand alone system
File room workstation
Hanging protocol
Navigation functions
Picture archiving and communication system (PACS)

Quality control (QC) station
Reading station
Review workstation
Softcopy
System architecture
Teleradiology
Web-based system
Workflow

The **picture archiving and communication system (PACS)** is becoming more commonplace in today's hospitals because hospital administrators have come to see the necessity of having such a system to serve physicians and patients even though the cost is great. The initial capital cost is great, but the benefit of having the system far outweighs the cost. This chapter outlines the basic concept of a PACS and its components, common PACS architecture, and typical PACS workflows that may be seen in a hospital.

FUNDAMENTALS

As discussed in Chapter 1, a PACS consists of digital acquisition, display workstations, and storage devices interconnected through an intricate network (Figure 8-1). The PACS is an electronic version of the radiologist reading room and the file room. The first PACSs were used in the early 1980s and generally served one single modality. Large research institutions housed early systems because most were developed by the scientists who worked at those institutions. As vendors became more involved, they developed proprietary systems that were very specific to their modalities. Finally, as physicians and hospitals became interested, it was determined that there must be standardization.

Digital imaging and communications in medicine (DICOM) is a universally accepted standard for exchanging medical images among the modality, viewing stations,

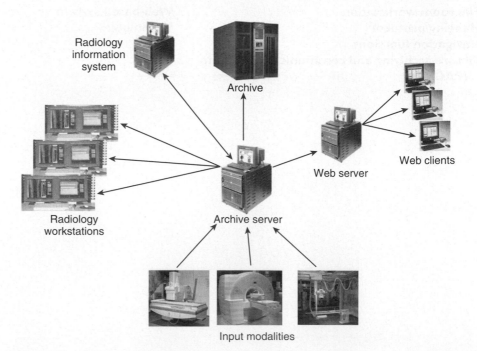

Figure 8-1 A typical PACS design.

and the archive. First completed in 1985, this standard laid the groundwork for the future development of integrated PACSs. Now each modality and PACS communicates via DICOM, and it continues to be refined every year. Every vendor and modality boasts DICOM compatibility (Figure 8-2), but each DICOM statement must be read carefully to determine the extent of the compatibility. DICOM compatibility issues are outside of the scope of this textbook.

To understand what a PACS is and how it is used, the following sections break down a PACS into its three fundamental parts (Figure 8-3): image acquisition, display workstations, and archive servers. Each of these topics is covered in depth in other chapters of the book.

Image Acquisition

In modern radiology departments, most images are acquired in a digital format, meaning that the images are inherently digital and can be transferred via a computer network. Ultrasound, computed tomography (CT), magnetic resonance imaging (MRI), and nuclear medicine have been digital for many years and have been taking advantage of PACS far longer than general radiography has. As stated earlier, the first PACS served a single modality, namely, ultrasound. Ultrasound mini-PACS networks were the norm in many hospitals. Radiologists routinely made diagnoses by looking at images on the modality's computer screen. It was a natural step from there to convert ultrasound to **softcopy** reporting, i.e., reading images on the computer without hardcopy films.

As the CT and MRI image sets became larger because of the increased number of cross-sectional images per patient, radiologists routinely went to the modality to view the images. This slowed down the scanning process for the technologists, and vendors began getting requests for extra console stations for radiologist viewing. These workstations were directly connected to the modalities. Radiologists could view the large stacks of images and perform simple image manipulation. These workstations morphed into mini-PACS and eventually into full-blown systems for CT and MRI. As discussed in Chapters 4 through 7, general radiography has taken the digital leap with computed radiography (CR) and direct and indirect capture digital radiography (DR). Now the conversion to a completely digital radiology department is a reality.

Display Workstations

A **display workstation** is any computer that a health care worker uses to view a digital image (Figure 8-4). It is the most interactive part of a PACS, and these workstations are used inside and outside of radiology. The display station receives images from the archive or from the various radiology modalities and presents them for viewing. The display workstation has PACS application software that allows the user to perform minor image-manipulation techniques to optimize the image being viewed. Some display stations have advanced software to perform more complex image-manipulation techniques. More details about display workstations will be given later in the chapter.

FUJIFILM

DICOM Conformance Statement

CR Console

(Standard)

April, 2004
5th Edition

Copyright Fuji Photo Film Co., Ltd., Japan

Figure 8-2 A DICOM conformance statement for a CT scanner.
(Courtesy Fuji Photo Film Co., Ltd., Tokyo, Japan.)

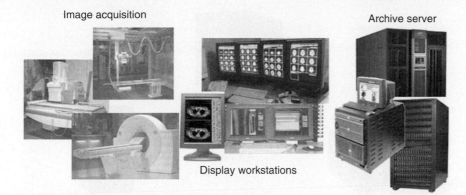

Figure 8-3 A collage of PACS components: image acquisition, display workstation, and archive server.

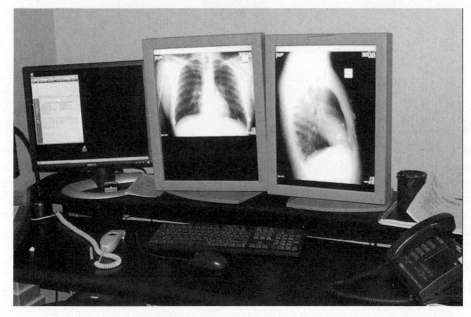

Figure 8-4 A display workstation for image review.

Archive Servers

An archive server is the file room of the PACS. It is composed of a database server or image manager, short-term and long-term storage, and a computer that controls the PACS workflow, known as a workflow manager (Figure 8-5). The **archive** is the central part of the PACS and houses all of the historic data along with the current data being generated. In many institutions the archive serves as the central hub that receives all images before being released to the radiologists for interpretation. The archive and all of its components will be studied in depth in Chapter 9.

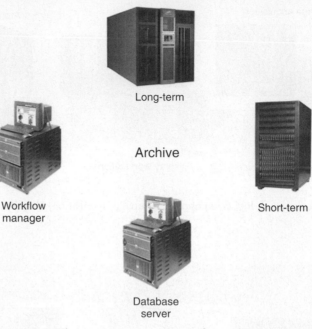

Figure 8-5 The common components of an archive.

Workflow

Workflow is a term that can be used in any industry or in any organization. It simply means how a process is done, step by step. In radiology, we have always used the term *workflow* to describe how we complete an examination from order entry to transcribed report. This section describes a generic film-based workflow and then compares it with a generic PACS workflow. The workflow in each radiology department is different because there are many variables.

Film-Based Workflow

Most departments were designed years ago for film and chemical processing. Pass boxes were built into walls that fed into darkrooms and into large open reading rooms that had gigantic multiviewer lightboxes lining the walls (see Figure 8-11). Eventually chemical processing time decreased from a few minutes to less than 60 seconds in some cases. As film and processing technology advanced, workflow became more efficient, despite having to still hand deliver film to radiologists and to make the occasional copy for a referring physician.

The following list outlines a typical workflow in a radiology department, from entering the order to transcribing the report (Figure 8-6).

■   The first step in any radiology department workflow is the entry of the order. The order may be a paper prescription from the ordering doctor, or the order may have been placed in the computer system by the emergency room (ER) or intensive care unit (ICU) staff. Either way, an order is placed in the radiology information

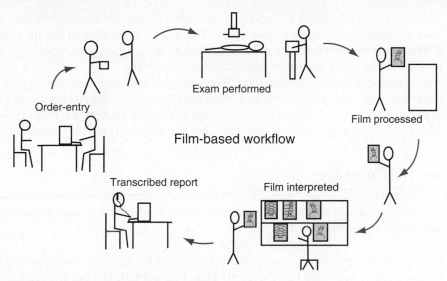

Order-entry

Exam performed

Film processed

Film-based workflow

Transcribed report

Film interpreted

Figure 8-6 A typical film-based workflow from order entry to transcribed report.

system (RIS), and a requisition is generated. A requisition generally contains the following information:

- Patient's name
- Patient's hospital identification (ID) number
- Date of birth
- Ordering physician's name
- Examination ordered
- Reason for examination
- Chief complaint

■ The paper requisition is then passed on to the technologist who will be performing the examination.

■ The technologist prepares the room for the patient and brings the patient back to the room.

■ The technologist verifies all of the patient's information and completes a patient history. The technologist also inquires whether the patient needs a complete set of copies to take to the next doctor's appointment.

■ The technologist performs the examination and processes all of the film after the complete examination is done.

■ The technologist critiques each film and repeats exposures as necessary.

■ The technologist makes copies if necessary and releases the patient with the films.

■ The technologist goes to the file room to find the film jacket with all of the patient's historic images, if applicable. The film jacket may not be located on site and may be kept at an off-site storage location. The film jacket is ordered to be picked up by the film courier.

■ The film jacket arrives a couple of hours or even days later, and the current films are hung on a multiviewer lightbox to be read by a radiologist. The file room clerk may hang a set of historic images from the film jacket for comparison.

■ The radiologist reads the films and dictates a report into the dictation system.

- The multiviewer lightbox is cleared of read films by the file room clerk, and the films are placed back into the film jacket. The film jacket is filed in the file room.
- A transcriptionist retrieves the recorded dictation and transcribes a report into the RIS. This may occur later that same day or the next day.
- The radiologist reviews the report, makes corrections, and signs the report as final. The final report is printed and placed in the patient's film jacket along with any previous reports. A final report is also sent to the ordering physician for review. This final report may come several days after the examination was completed.

Generic PACS Workflow

The PACS workflow is in many ways different from the film-based workflow (Figure 8-7). The technologist may get the order via an electronic worklist or a paper requisition, but after that, things begin to change.

- Changes in the order entry are on the horizon, but for now, the order-entry process is the same as in film-based departments. The technologist needs a requisition to verify the patient ID and to take a patient history.
- The order is input into the RIS, and the RIS sends a message to the PACS to find all historic images and put them on the short-term archive. This eliminates waiting for the file room to retrieve a film jacket from the off-site storage location.
- The technologist prepares the room, retrieves the patient, and performs the patient history. The history is recorded on the paper requisition or input electronically into the patient's computerized medical record.
- The technologist performs the examination, and depending on the type of image acquisition device, the images are processed and repeated as necessary and sent to the appropriate PACS device. The patient images have been tagged with informa-

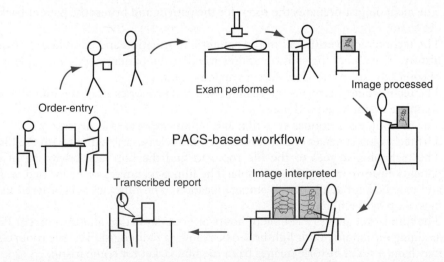

Figure 8-7 This diagram represents a typical PACS-based workflow from order entry to transcribed report.

tion from the RIS so that historic image reports are available at the PACS when the new images are sent.

■ The requisition is either taken to the radiologist, or the radiologist may pull the images from an electronic worklist. The radiologist also pulls up historic images and reports and compares the previous images with the current images.

■ The radiologist dictates a report and has it transcribed, or voice recognition software may be used. If the radiologist uses voice recognition software, he or she can review the report right after dictation, make corrections, and sign the report, making it final.

With PACS it is possible that the time it takes from performing the examination to completing the final radiologist's report is only a couple hours, compared with a couple days for the film-based workflow.

SYSTEM ARCHITECTURE

System architecture can be defined as the hardware and software infrastructure of a computer system. In a PACS, the system architecture normally consists of acquisition devices, storage, display workstations, and an image management system. The following discussion outlines three common PACS architectures and takes a look at the flow of images after acquisition.

Client/Server-Based Systems

In a **client/server-based system,** images are sent directly to the archive server after acquisition and are centrally located (Figure 8-8). The display workstation functions as a client of the archive server and accesses images based on a centralized worklist that is generated at the archive server. The health care worker at the display workstation chooses a name from the central list, and the archive server sends the image data to display station. After the "client" is finished, the image data are flushed from its memory. Most systems allow basic image manipulation at the display workstation or "client," and the changes are saved on the archive server.

Advantages

■ Any examination sent to the PACS is available anywhere without other interventions.
■ Only one person can open the study with the intent to read it. Others that open the study will receive a message that the study is open and being read.
■ There is no need to pull or send historic images to a particular workstation because the old studies are available with the new on the archive.

Disadvantages

■ The archive server is seen as a single point of failure. If the archive goes down, the entire system is down, and no image movement can take place. All newly acquired images must remain at the modality until the archive is up and can again receive the images.

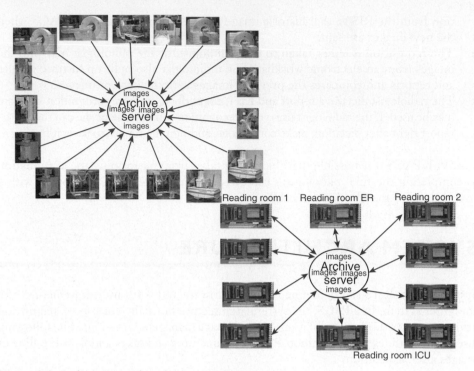

Figure 8-8 A client/server-based system architecture.

- The system is very network dependent. The images are flying back and forth between the archive and the workstations, and the network can become bogged down because of the large volume of data being moved.
- The archive server is handling many requests at once and can become bottlenecked because of the high volume of requests.

Distributed Systems

In a **distributed or stand-alone system,** the acquisition modalities send the images to a designated reading station and possibly to review stations, depending on where the order originated (i.e., ICU or ER) (Figure 8-9). In some systems, the images are sent from the modality to the archive server, and the archive server distributes the images to the designated workstation. The reading station designations may be designed based on radiologist reading preferences. For example, MRI may be sent to one station and CT to another, or all cross-sectional neurological images may be sent to one station but all body imaging are sent to another. The designation is decided after extensive workflow observation. Moreover, in a distributed model, the workstations can query and retrieve images from the archive. All images are then stored locally and then are sent to the archive server after they have been read. These images remain on the local hard drive of the workstation until they are deleted either by a user or by system rules.

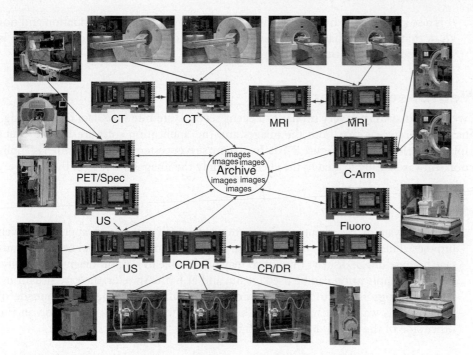

Figure 8-9 A distributed system architecture model.

Advantages

■ If the archive server goes down, local reading at the workstations is not interrupted, other than not being able to get historic images. After the archive comes back up, the images that have been changed and signed off by the radiologist will be forwarded automatically to the archive to be saved.

■ Because the images can be distributed to many locations at once, copies of an examination exist at various locations. Therefore it is less likely that PACS data will be lost.

■ The system is less dependent on the network for its speed. The user can be working on one examination while the workstation is pulling and getting the next examination ready to be read. The workstation can fetch historic images according to rules the user sets up.

Disadvantages

■ There is heavy reliance on the assumption that the distribution of images is being done correctly. If the distribution is wrong, the prefetching of historic examinations will not be correct either.

■ Each workstation has a different worklist, and therefore only one person can be working on that list at a time.

■ It can be inconvenient to read additional studies; the radiologist would have to move to another workstation to read the images designated for that workstation.

■ The users must depend on the query-and-retrieve function when nonscheduled examinations arrive at the workstation to be read.

■ It is also possible for two radiologists to be reading the same examination and not know that the other has it until they try to start dictation. The paper requisition is very important with this type of PACS.

Web-Based Systems

A **web-based system** is very similar to a client/server system in how data flow. The significant difference is that both the images and the application software for the client display are held centrally (Figure 8-10). In a client/server system, the client still has application software locally loaded to the client, and only the images are held at the archive.

Advantages

■ The hardware at the client can be anything that will support an appropriate web browser. This allows for greater flexibility with hardware but can also be a disadvantage because image displays (monitors) may not be able to support diagnostic quality.
■ The same application can be used on site and at home in teleradiology situations. **Teleradiology** is a term used to describe the reading of images from outside of the hospitals walls. It can be down the road at the radiologist's home or on the other side of the world during nighttime hours.

Disadvantages

■ The system's functionality may be limited because the software is not installed locally. The bandwidth of the network connection limits the amount of data that can be transmitted for download, and some programs are too large to be transmitted over the network that is installed.
■ As with client/server systems, the network is the biggest obstacle to performance.

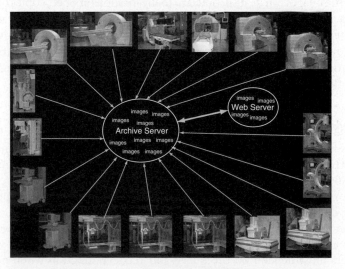

Figure 8-10 A web-based system architecture.

DISPLAY WORKSTATIONS

The display workstation is the most interactive part of a PACS, consisting of a monitor and a computer with a mouse and keyboard. In addition, each system has hardware that fits the users' requirements.

As you know, conventional film/screen radiography uses large multiviewer light-boxes to display the images (Figure 8-11). Early in the history of PACS, radiologists believed that they needed four to six monitors to match the viewing capability they had with the lightboxes. As the radiologists have become more comfortable viewing images on monitors, the number of monitors required by the radiologists has decreased to an average of two (Figure 8-12). This decrease can also be attributed in part to the continued development of viewing software and better hardware, namely, mice.

The monitor is one of the most important elements of a PACS display station. The cathode ray tube (CRT) (Figure 8-13) and the liquid crystal display (LCD) (Figure 8-14) are the most popular types of monitors in a radiology department. The LCD has decreased in price and increased in quality during the past few years and will soon take over the entire PACS display market because of its size, resolution, and lack of heat production. The LCD also requires less maintenance, gives out more light, and can be used in areas with a high amount of ambient light. In early PACS reading rooms, supplemental air conditioning had to be installed to offset the heat put out by multiple CRTs. Along with the number of monitors used, the

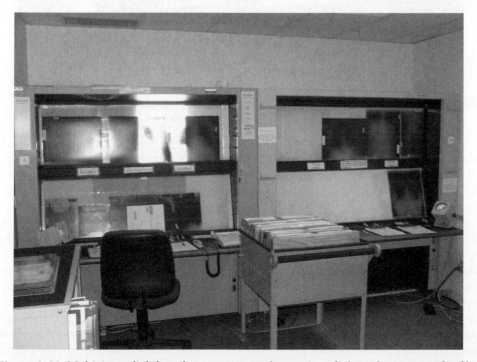

Figure 8-11 Multiviewer lightbox that was commonly seen in radiology departments for film viewing.

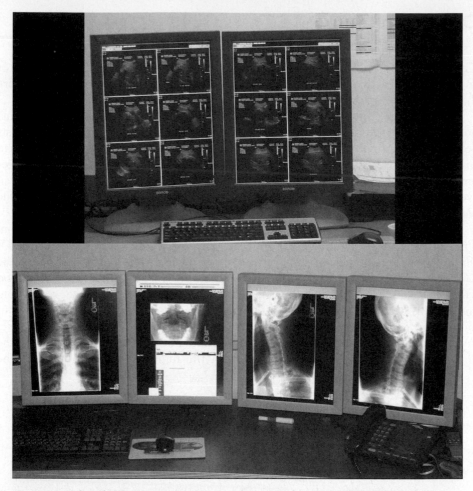

Figure 8-12 A four-bank monitor workstation and a two-bank monitor workstation.

resolution and orientation of the monitor are also factors in determining which type of monitor to buy for each workstation. Most cross-sectional imaging is read on a 1K square monitor (Figure 8-15), and most CR and DR are read on at least a 2K portrait monitor (Figure 8-16).

Remember from Chapter 2 that a basic picture element on a display is known as a pixel. The number of pixels contained on a display is known as its resolution. The relationship between pixels and resolution can be stated as follows: the more pixels in an image, the higher the resolution of the image, and the more information that can be displayed. Resolution can also be defined as the process or capability of distinguishing between individual parts of an image that are adjacent. Pixels are arranged in a matrix. A matrix is a rectangular or square table of numbers that represents the pixel intensity to be displayed on the monitor. Common screen resolutions that are found on today's monitors are 1280 × 1024 (1K), 1600 × 1200 (2K), 2048 × 1536 (3K), and 2048 × 2560 (5K).

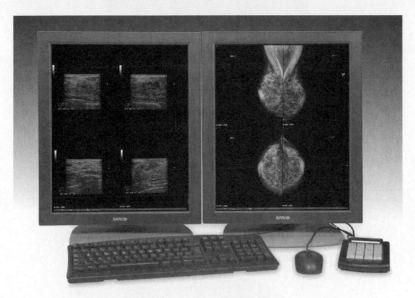

Figure 8-13 A cathode ray tube (CRT) monitor.
(Courtesy Agfa, Mortsel, Belgium.)

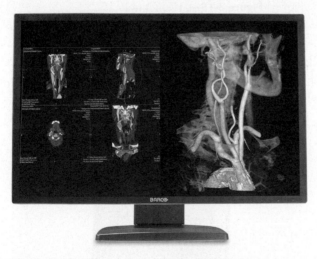

Figure 8-14 A liquid crystal display (LCD) monitor.
(Courtesy Barco, Kortrijk, Belgium.)

Medical displays are generally of a higher quality than displays used for other applications. Radiologists often use the highest resolution monitors available for the modality that is being read. For example, mammography requires a 5K or 5-megapixel resolution to provide the viewing capacity needed, but a cross-sectional image requires only a 1K monitor to view the necessary information. Because a referring physician is not the primary doctor reading the examinations, a 1K monitor would be sufficient for his or her viewing needs.

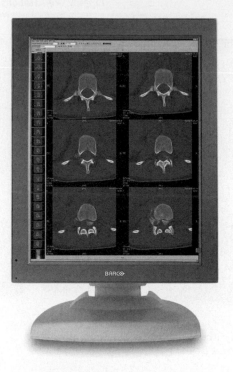

Figure 8-15 A 1K monitor.
(Courtesy Barco.)

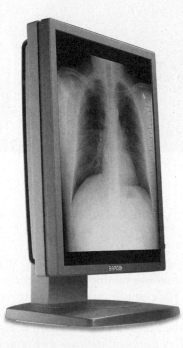

Figure 8-16 A 2K monitor.
(Courtesy Barco.)

Display stations can be categorized by their primary use: primary reading stations for radiologists, review stations for referring physicians, technologist quality control (QC) stations where technologists review images, and image management stations for the file room personnel. Each of these workstations has one specific main purpose and is strategically located near the end-user of its designated purpose.

Radiologist Reading Stations

The radiologist **reading station** (Figure 8-17) is used by a radiologist when making a primary diagnosis. The reading station has the highest quality hardware, including the best monitor. The computer hardware meets the needs of the PACS vendor, but it will usually be very robust, requiring little downtime. The keyboard and mouse can be customized. There are many different styles of mice available that can increase the efficiency of the software being used (Figure 8-18).

There is generally access to a nearby RIS, with a dictation system near or even connected to the PACS station. Many PACSs have software that integrates the RIS and dictation system.

Physician Review Stations

The physician **review workstation** (Figure 8-19) is a step-down model of the radiologist reading station. Many vendors use the same level of software but may eliminate some of the more advanced functions. One of the most important features on a physician review station is the ability to view current and previous reports along with

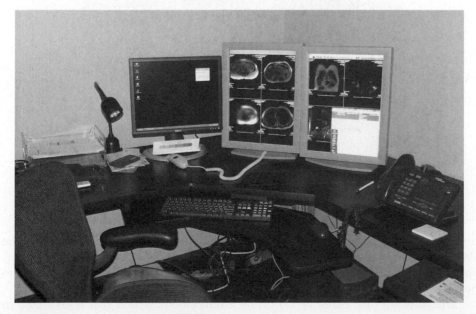

Figure 8-17 A radiologist reading station.

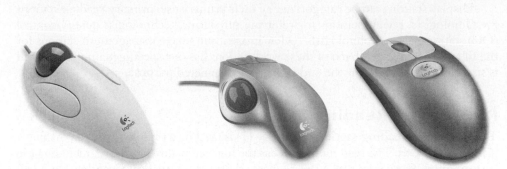

Figure 8-18 A wheel mouse, trackball mouse, and an ergonomic mouse.
(Courtesy Logitech, Fremont, CA.)

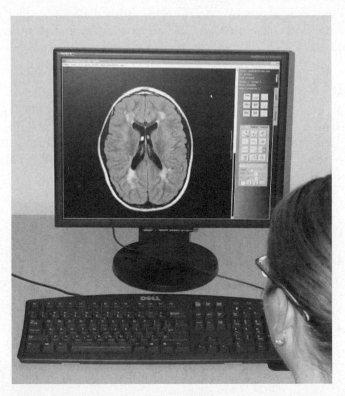

Figure 8-19 A physician review station.

the images. This can be accomplished with the integration of RIS functions with the PACS software mentioned above. Most referring physicians want to read the radiologist's report along with seeing the patient's images, and often the report is more important to them than the images.

The software may either be loaded on a stand-alone station that is dedicated to viewing images, or it may be delivered over a web browser on any personal computer (PC) within an office or on a floor. In high-volume areas such as the ER and ICU

(Figure 8-20), there are dedicated PACS workstations for image viewing. These dedicated stations may have the higher-end monitors like the radiologist reading stations, but many may have lower-end monitors because of cost constraints.

One of the greatest advantages of a PACS is the ability to view the same set of images in multiple locations at one time. In the film/screen era, referring physicians would make the trek to the radiology department to consult with a radiologist about a patient's image, hoping that the films would be found in the file room and that the radiologist was available to consult. Now with PACS, the referring physician can pull up the patient's images in his or her office and read the radiologist's report. The referring physician and the radiologist can consult on the telephone while looking at the images simultaneously. This is one way that PACSs have improved continuity and speed of patient care.

Technologist QC Stations

The technologist **QC station** (Figure 8-21) is used to review images after acquisition but before sending them to the radiologist. The QC station may be used to improve or adjust image quality characteristics, or it may be used to verify patient demographic

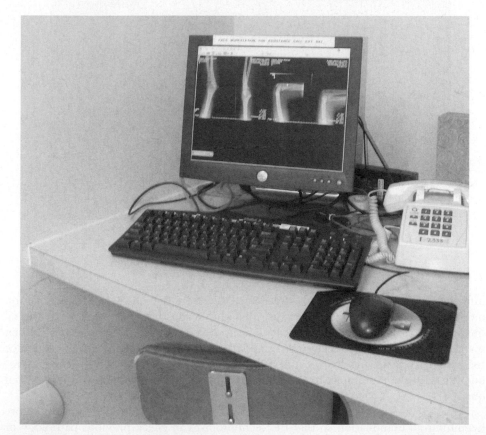

Figure 8-20 A physician review workstation.

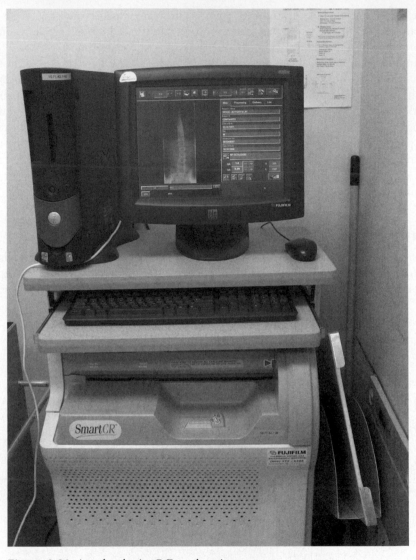

Figure 8-21 A technologist QC workstation.

information. Many QC stations are placed between the CR and DR acquisition modalities as a pass-through to ensure that the images have met the departmental quality standard. The technologist QC station generally has a 1K monitor. When manipulating images, the technologist must be careful not to change the appearance too much from the original acquired image. The technologist should consult frequently with the radiologist to ensure that the images being sent are of the required quality.

The QC workstation can also be used to query and retrieve historic images before beginning an examination so that the technologist can check previous pathology or body characteristics. This can help with the selection of technical factors or procedural protocol. It is common protocol in a film-based department to pull film jackets on patients before performing an examination. The QC station affords the same benefit as pulling the film jacket.

File Room/Image Management Stations

The file room in a PACS environment has seen many changes in the past few years. Before PACS, the file room was a large open room with endless rows of shelves full of film jackets. Today a file room in a PACS environment may be as simple as a couple of computers and a dry laser to make copies for outside needs.

The **file room workstation** (Figure 8-22) may be used to look up examinations for a physician or to print copies of images for the patient to take to an outside physician. Many hospitals are moving away from printing films to save the cost of the film and are instead moving toward burning compact disks (CDs) with the patient's images because they are less expensive. The CD of images can be viewed on any PC and generally comes with easy-to-use software burned onto it with the images.

The file room may also be responsible for correcting patient demographics. If images with incorrect demographics are sent to the archive, then it is difficult to pull those images the next time the patient comes in for an examination. The archive is a database and is only as good as the information that is put into it.

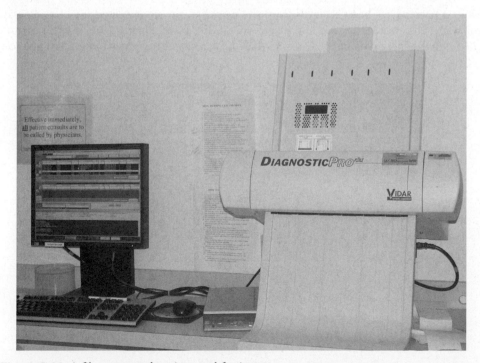

Figure 8-22 A file room workstation used for image management purposes.

Common Functions

This section provides an overview of common functions found on a PACS workstation. All of the functions should be available on any level of the workstation except for the advanced functions, which are specific to different types of workstations. The functions can be broken down into four categories: navigation functions, image manipulation and enhancement functions, image management functions, and advanced workstation functions.

Navigation Functions

Navigation functions (Figure 8-23) are used to move through images, series, studies, and patients. The worklist is used to navigate through patients. Most worklists are customizable for the user. One doctor may want to see only unread CT studies, and another may want to see all neurologic studies done that day regardless of the modality. Most modern PACS software conforms to the Windows (Microsoft, Redmond, WA) look and feel. The use of grab bars on the right side of Windows to scroll through a list and the activation of the scroll wheel on the mouse to scroll through the list are common features. The mouse is also a very useful navigation tool. The right mouse offers many short-cut features in a menu of frequently used tasks and applications.

Hanging Protocols

Once a patient has been selected from the worklist, the images load into the display software. In most PACSs, each user has the ability to set up custom hanging protocols. A **hanging protocol** (Figure 8-24) is how a set of images will be displayed on

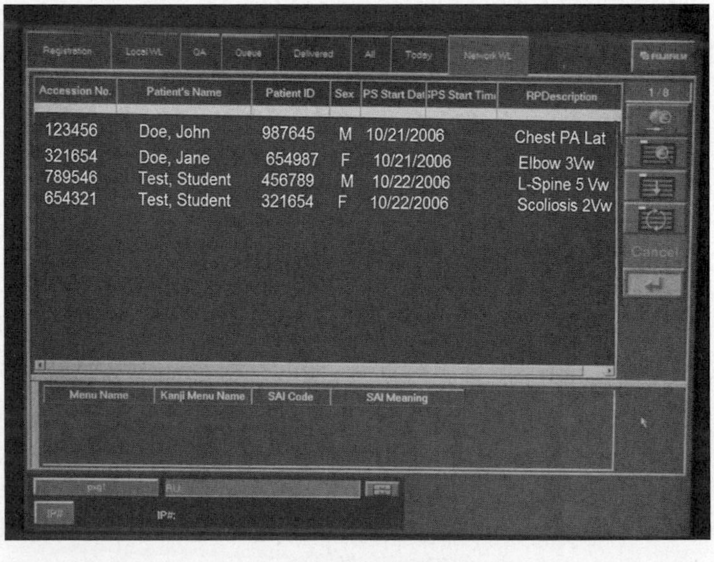

Figure 8-23 A screen shot of PACS worklist.

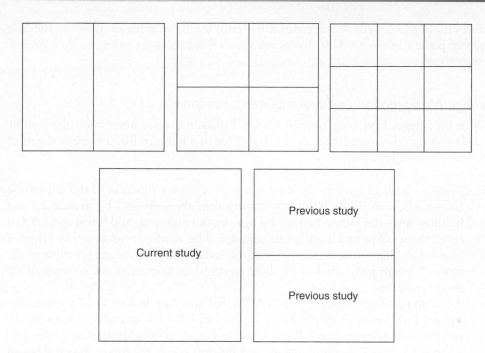

Figure 8-24 Typical hanging protocols seen on a PACS workstation.

the monitor. For example, when I select a CT examination, I want to view four images on each monitor, but when I view a CR image, I want to view one image on each monitor.

Users can choose the hanging protocols they prefer for each modality. The hanging protocols can also be required to show the previous examination on one monitor and the current examination on the other. Once the hanging protocols have been set, the most efficient study navigation is determined.

Study Navigation

A *study* in PACS is the current or previous examination being viewed. A study may comprise two or three single images such as the case with CR and DR, or it may contain several series of images such as the case with MRI. The images can be paged through either with the scroll wheel or with arrows on the keyboard, or they can be run through in stacks. Many vendors call the stack mode of scrolling through images *cine*. This term comes from the word *cinematic*, and it means *to move through frame by frame of the series of images*. The images can be quickly moved through manually using the mouse, but most vendors have an automatic setting that runs through the images at a preset pace. The cine function is used most often in cross-sectional imaging.

Many vendors provide icons (pictures within the software that activate software functions) that allow the user to move among a patient's various studies or open the next unread patient in the worklist after having read the current study. Another navigation tool that is commonly found is a close patient or close study icon. This icon closes the active patient or study and either pulls up the worklist or moves to the next unread patient in the worklist. Users can set up these tools according to their preferences.

Image Manipulation and Enhancement Functions

Once the images have been opened on the display, there are many tools that can be used to change the appearance of the image. Here is a bulleted list of some of the most commonly used functions:

- Window/level (Figure 8-25): This is usually a default function of the left mouse button when an image is actively displayed in the software. By depressing and holding down the mouse button and moving the mouse up and down and left and right, the window and level can be adjusted. The window represents the range of gray values that are being viewed, and the level represents the center value of the range. Changing the window and level changes the brightness and contrast of the image on screen.
- Annotations (Figure 8-26): Most PACSs can annotate text or graphics onto the image. This function should NOT be used to label left or right to indicate the patient's side because digital R and L will not hold up in court because of the ability to mark anywhere on the image and flip and rotate the image into any layout on the screen. Annotations can indicate prone or supine, 30 minutes, upright or flat, or any other image information the department deems appropriate. Radiologists frequently place arrows or circles around pathology or questionable areas so that the referring physician can pinpoint what is in question.
- Flip and rotate (Figure 8-27): These functions are used to orient the image in the anatomical hanging position desired by the department. There are usually left-to-

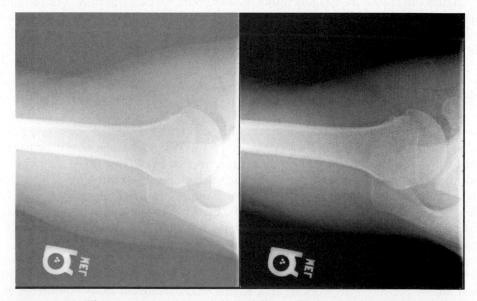

Figure 8-25 The same image, but each has a different window/level setting.

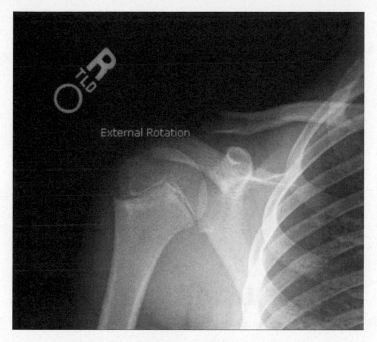

Figure 8-26 Text annotations can be placed directly on the image.

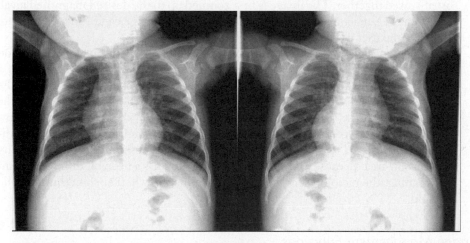

Figure 8-27 This image has been flipped left to right.

right flip and 90-degree clockwise and counterclockwise icons. This function makes it very important that lead markers are used to ensure that the radiologist reads the correct side.

■ Pan, zoom, and magnify (Figure 8-28): These functions are used primarily by the radiologist to increase the size of an area on the image. The magnify function will usually enlarge a square area of the image, and the square can be moved around the image to quickly see various areas enlarged. The pan and zoom functions are

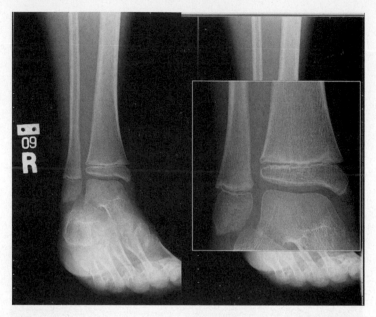

Figure 8-28 This section of the image has been magnified to show closer detail of the bone.

usually used together. The image is first zoomed up to the desired magnified level, and then the pan icon is activated so that the zoomed image can be moved around, allowing the user to view the different areas of the image.

- Measurements (Figure 8-29): There are various measurement functions found on a PACS station. The most common is the distance measurement. The size of a pixel is a known measurement, so the software can measure structures on the image based on this known measurement. Another common measurement is the angle measurement, which measures the angle between two structures. It is commonly used when reading spine studies. Another common measurement a radiologist may use is a region of interest (ROI). It will determine the pixel intensity of a certain area. Because each type of tissue or fluid has a little bit different intensity reading, the radiologist can make a determination whether something is solid or fluid.

Image Management Functions

Most PACSs allow the user to modify patient demographics (Figure 8-30) at the technologist QC station, the reading station, and the file room station. It is imperative that the patient demographics are correct. If wrong information is archived, images will not come up when correct information is entered when trying to retrieve them. Only make changes when the information is absolutely known to be wrong. To minimize errors, many hospitals only allow certain people the access to change demographics.

Another image management function is the query/retrieve function used to retrieve studies from the archive (Figure 8-31). The query function allows the user to

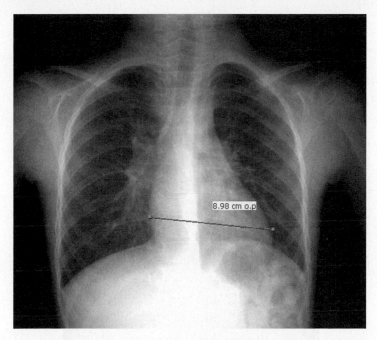

Figure 8-29 The distance measurement tool can be used to measure structures on the image.

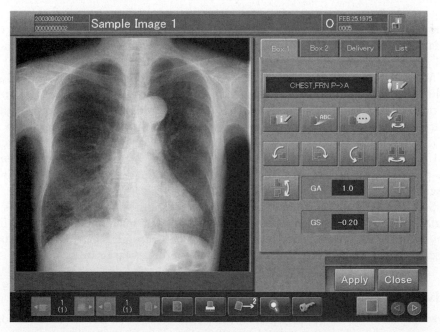

Figure 8-30 Patient demographics can be changed after image acquisition on some PACS workstations.
(Courtesy Fuji.)

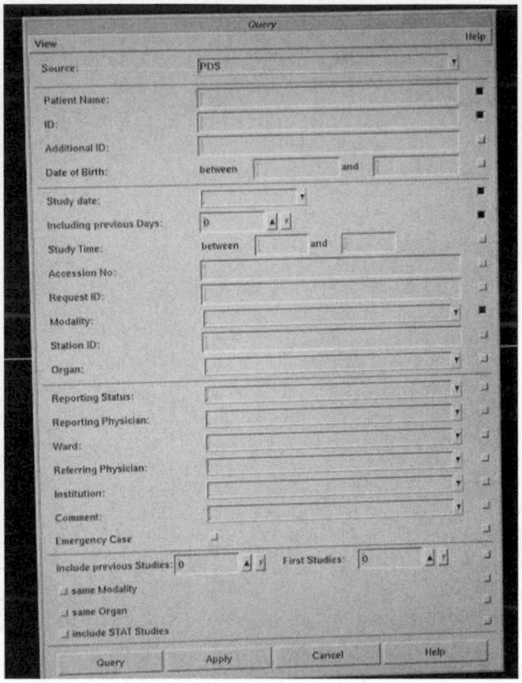

Figure 8-31 The user can query images from the archive using various search parameters.

query a study on multiple fields such as the patient's name or ID, date of service, or modality. Some systems also allow a query based on a diagnosis code or comment field.

Many vendors have provided a CD-burning option that allows users to save studies to a CD for outside use. The feature may only be available in the file room to control the CDs that are sent out. Health Insurance Portability and Accountability Act (HIPAA) compliance must also be maintained. Another common feature is the ability to copy and paste images into a document. This is frequently used with the web-based systems when creating presentations for conferences. The patient information must be removed from the image before it is placed into a presentation.

Some hospitals have retained the ability to print films for outside use. This is also usually done only in the file room so that control can be maintained over the printed films for HIPAA purposes and cost reasons. Some hospitals have also connected workstations to paper printers for quick consults and medical records.

Advanced Workstation Functions

Advanced functions are usually placed on specialty workstations for the radiologist, but some are found on the technologist QC station to further enhance the images. Here is a bulleted list of some of the most common advanced functions.

Reading Station Advanced Functions

- Multiplanar reconstruction (MPR) (Figure 8-32): One of the most commonly used three-dimensional (3D) rendering techniques. When doing a CT scan of a patient, thin axial slices can be acquired of a volume of tissue. The slices can then be loaded into the MPR software, and a reconstruction in another plane can be produced. The most common application is producing coronal images from the axial set to reduce radiation to the patient and scan time at the modality.

- Maximum intensity projection and minimum intensity projection (MIP and MinIp) (Figure 8-33): Used to visualize vessels (MIP) and air-filled structures (MinIp). Commonly performed after the injection of contrast on CT and MRI studies, the contrast will show areas of strictures and blockages within the vessels.

- Volume rendering technique (VRT) (Figure 8-34): Similar to MIP but allows the user to assign colors based on the intensity of the tissue so that bone, contrast agent, and organs can be seen in different colors. The technique uses a histogram-type graph to differentiate the various structures.

- Shaded surface display (SSD) (Figure 8-35): Using a threshold of pixel intensity values, everything below the threshold will be removed, and everything above will be assigned a color and shown as a 3D object.

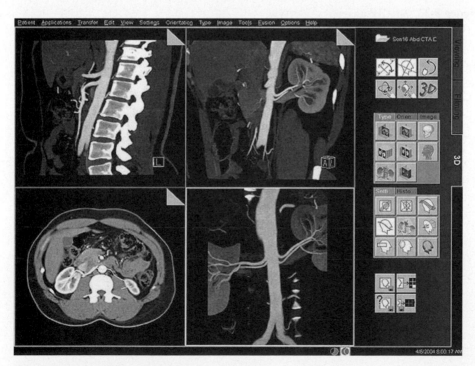

Figure 8-32 An MPR image.
(Courtesy Siemens, Berlin and Munich, Germany.)

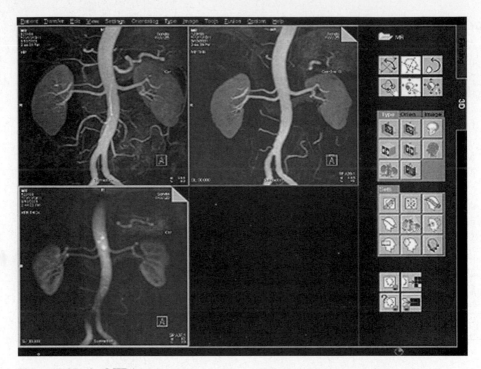

Figure 8-33 An MIP image.
(Courtesy Siemens.)

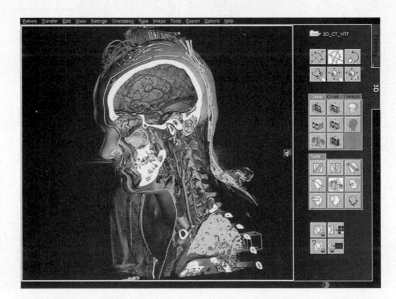

Figure 8-34 A VRT image.
(Courtesy Siemens.)

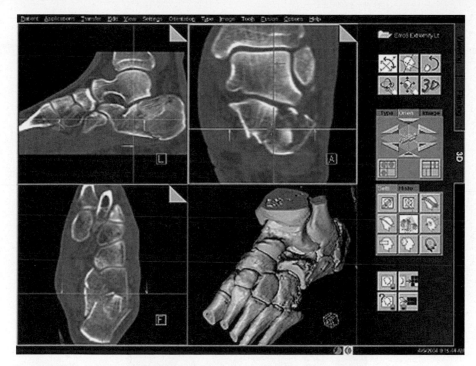

Figure 8-35 A 3D shaded surface image.
(Courtesy Siemens.)

Technologist QC Station Advanced Functions

■ Stitching (Figure 8-36): Used when multiple images need to be put together into one image. The most common application is for full-spine x-rays or a scoliosis series. The examination was traditionally performed on a 3-foot film and processed; CR manufacturers have developed a 3-foot CR cassette that contains multiple imaging plates (IPs). Each of the IPs is scanned through the reader, and the individual images are sent to the QC workstation. The software then interpolates the images and connects them using known markers from the IPs. The technologist can adjust how the images are connected. Another application of stitching is producing long leg images for leg length discrepancy studies. The images are acquired in a fashion similar to the one described above and stitched together. If the special 3-foot cassettes are not available, a radiopaque ruler must be used to ensure that the images are stitched at the right area.

■ Image postprocessing: Is regarded as an advanced function of the workstation.

There are many other advanced workstation functions available to be added to the PACS workstation. This is a growing field with advancements coming each year. Specific information about how to perform these procedures can be found in the vendor's user manual.

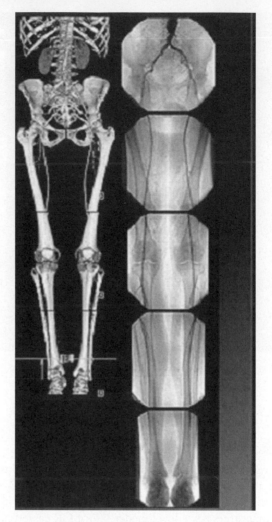

Figure 8-36 This image was stitched together from two separate images.
(Courtesy Siemens.)

SUMMARY

- A PACS consists of digital acquisition, display workstations, and storage devices interconnected through an intricate network.
- DICOM is a universally accepted standard for exchanging medical images between the modality, viewing stations, and the archive.
- A display workstation is any computer that a health care worker uses to view a digital image, and it is the most interactive part of a PACS.
- The archive is the central part of the PACS and houses all of the historic data along with the current data being generated.

- Workflow is how a process is done step by step or how a task is completed.
- System architecture can be defined as the hardware and software infrastructure of a computerized system.
- Common system architectures found with a PACS are client/server-based systems, distributed or stand-alone systems, and web-based systems.
- Display stations can be categorized by their primary use, such as reading stations for radiologists, review stations for referring physicians, technologist QC station for technologist review of images, and image management station for the file room personnel.
- There are many functions available on a PACS workstation, and each set of functions can be broken down into four categories: navigation functions, image manipulation and enhancement functions, image management functions, and advanced workstation functions.

CHAPTER REVIEW QUESTIONS

1. What does the acronym PACS stand for, and what is its definition?

2. What are the different types of PACS workstations, and how are they used?

3. Define workflow, and give an example of a generic PACS workflow from scheduled procedure to finalized report.

4. What is the definition of system architecture, and what are the three major models?

5. What are the advantages and disadvantages of the three system architecture models?

6. What are the most common functions found on a PACS workstation?

7. What specialized PACS workstations may be found in a hospital, and how are they used?

CHAPTER 9

PACS Archiving

Archiving Components

Image Manager
Image Storage

Archive Considerations

1. Describe the use of an image archive.
2. Explain the function of the image manager.
3. Discuss the uses of short-term archive storage.
4. Describe the levels 0, 1, 3, and 5 of redundant array of independent disks.
5. Compare and contrast the various long-term archive technologies used in current picture archival and communication systems.
6. Define the concept of an application service provider.

KEY TERMS

Application service provider (ASP)
Archive
Archive server
Digital versatile disk (DVD)
Disaster recovery
Image manager
Image storage

Magnetic disk storage
Magneto-optical disk (MOD)
Redundant array of independent (inexpensive) disks (RAID)
Tape
Tier
Ultra density optical (UDO) disk

ARCHIVING COMPONENTS

The term **archive** can be defined as a place where records or documents are preserved (Figure 9-1). In a picture archival and communication system (PACS), the electronic archive serves as the new file room and warehouse for all digital imaging and communications in medicine (DICOM) imaging modalities (Figure 9-2). It stores all patient and image data, often on magnetic tape or optical disk. The PACS archive controls the receipt, storage, and distribution of new and historic images. With the explosion of digital imaging in radiology, the archive is one of the fastest growing components in the PACS. Archive technology continues to make drastic improvements each year; the storage capacity is said to double every 18 to 24 months, and the price per gigabyte also continues to decrease.

The archive is a complex arrangement of computers and storage space. As a whole, it consists of several components, both hardware and software. These can be divided into two major categories: image manager/controller and image storage/server or

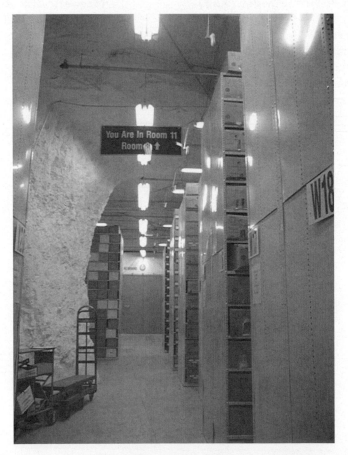

Figure 9-1 The archives at the National Archives in Washington, DC.

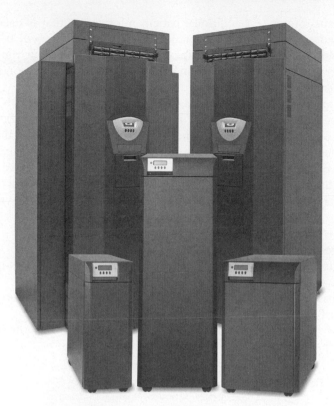

Figure 9-2 MOD and jukebox.
(Courtesy Sun Microsystems.)

archive server. The next two sections discuss image management and image storage. Various types of image storage hardware are described. The chapter ends with a discussion of things to consider when choosing an archiving system.

Image Manager

The **image manager** contains the master database of everything that is in the archive. It controls the receipt, retrieval, and distribution of the images it stores and also controls all the DICOM processes running within the archive.

The image manager generally runs a reliable commercial database such as Sybase (Sybase Inc., Dublin, CA) or Oracle (Oracle Corp., Redwood Shores, CA) with structured query language (SQL). This database contains only the image header information, not the image data. The image data are stored on the archive server, which will be discussed in the next section. The database is mirrored, meaning that there are two identical databases running simultaneously so that if one goes down, the system can call on the mirror and continue to run as normal, a very important feature.

The image manager is also the PACS component that interfaces with the radiology information system (RIS) and the hospital information system (HIS). This allows the PACS database to collect additional patient information that is necessary for its effective operation. Information extracted from these databases will be used in the prefetching and routing of images to various locations throughout the PACS. The image manager can also play a key role in populating image information into the hospital electronic medical record (EMR).

As mentioned earlier, the image manager database contains the DICOM header information, such as the patient name, identification information (ID), examination date, ordering physician, and location. These fields are organized within the database so that when someone queries for a study on a workstation, the image manager can quickly move through these data fields and locate the images that are being queried (Figure 9-3). The database has pointers associated with each image on the archive server that point back to the data fields within the database. The following list summarizes the process:

- An order is placed in the RIS for a radiology study.
- The images are acquired and sent to the archive.
- The image manager strips the image header from each image and assigns a pointer to each image or series of images.
- The database files the information in various fields and communicates back to the RIS to verify certain information.
- The study is then queried, and the pointers locate the images on the archive server and send the images to the workstation.

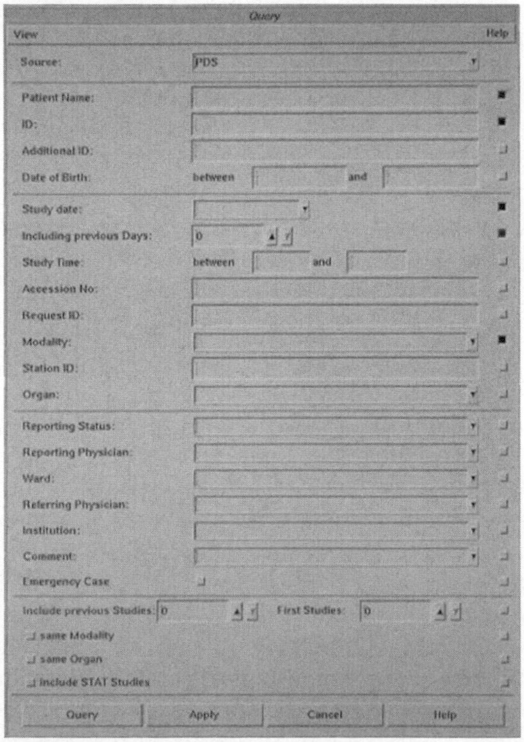

Figure 9-3 The PACS database can be queried using various data points.

Image Storage

The **image storage** or **archive server** consists of the physical storage device of the archive system. It commonly consists of two or three tiers of storage. A **tier** is a level, layer, or division of something. In an archive server, a tier represents a specific level of archive: short term, mid term, or long term. Most PACS archive systems are set up with a short-term tier and a long-term tier. Short-term means being online or available very quickly, usually within 3 to 5 seconds. Long-term means near line, or images that must be retrieved from a tape or disk storage device and brought to redundant array of independent disks (RAIDs). This could take 1 to 5 minutes.

Short-Term Storage

The short-term tier is commonly a **redundant array of independent (inexpensive) disks (RAID)** (Figure 9-4). A RAID is composed of several magnetic disks or hard drives that are linked together in an array (Figure 9-5). The size of the RAID ranges

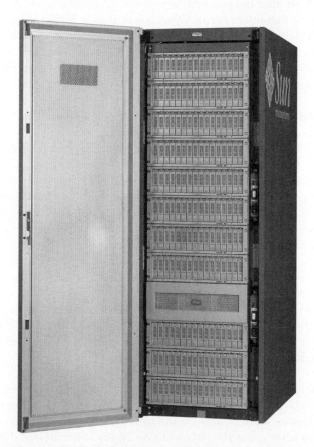

Figure 9-4 A redundant array of independent disks.
(Courtesy Sun Microsystems.)

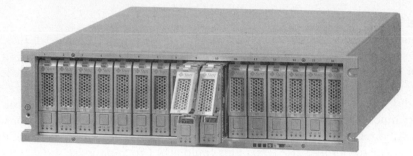

Figure 9-5 A RAID array.
(Courtesy Sun Microsystems.)

from several hundred gigabytes to several terabytes. As the individual disk sizes continue to increase, so does the potential size of the RAID.

In 1988 David Patterson, Garth Gibson, and Randy Katz coined the term RAID in an article entitled "A Case for Redundant Arrays of Inexpensive Disks (RAID)." Their presentation introduced five levels of RAID; now there are approximately 11 levels (Figure 9-6), most of which are combinations of the first five. Four RAID levels that are most commonly used:

- RAID 0: Data are "striped" across all of the connected disks. "Striping" means that the data are broken up into pieces, and each disk will have one piece of the data (Figure 9-7). When the data are called up from the RAID, all of the data are put together from the disks and presented to the user as a whole.
- RAID 1: All of the data sent to the RAID are mirrored onto two disks (Figure 9-8). Mirroring means that all of the data are duplicated and placed onto two separate disks. This RAID level has full redundancy, meaning that if one disk goes down, the other one takes over and operation of the system continues. This is a very expensive system because only half of the total storage is used.
- RAID 3: The data are striped across all of the disks just like in RAID 0, but there is one disk that is set aside for error correction. This disk is known as the parity disk (Figure 9-9).
- RAID 5: This RAID level is similar to RAID 3 but instead of having the parity written to one disk, it is striped along all of the disks within the RAID (Figure 9-10). RAID 5 is the most common level used for a PACS archive because it provides adequate redundancy and fault tolerance.

The striping of data increases the reliability and performance of the system. With certain levels of RAID, if one disk fails, the data from that disk can be regenerated using the redundancy of data on the other disks. The error correction detects any transmission errors, and the data will also be regenerated based on the information from the other disks. Striping also enhances performance because if all of the data were on one disk, data added to the disk first would be accessed first, requiring

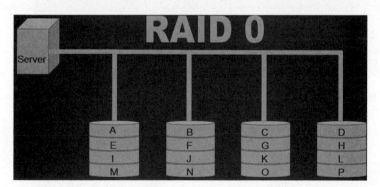

RAID 0	Striped – no fault tolerance
RAID 1	Mirroring
RAID 2	Error Correcting Coding
RAID 3	Byte level striping & dedicated parity
RAID 4	Block level striping & dedicated parity
RAID 5	Byte level striping & parity
RAID 6	Block-level striping with two parity blocks
RAID 10	Stripe of mirrors
RAID 0+1	Mirror of stripes
RAID 30	Striping of dedicated parity arrays
RAID 100	A stripe of RAID 10s
RAID 7, S, Z, 1.5	Proprietary

Figure 9-6 RAID levels.

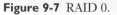

Figure 9-7 RAID 0.

longer wait times for data added to the disk later. Spreading data over several disks allows all data to be accessed at the same time.

Long-Term Storage

Because RAID is becoming more cost-effective, many hospitals use RAID storage for both their short-term and their long-term archive. Other long-term storage products that are still widely used are optical disk, tape, and magnetic disk. Optical disk and magnetic tape archive solutions use a jukebox (Figure 9-11) to hold the tapes or disks; the magnetic disk uses an array. The jukebox has controller software that interfaces

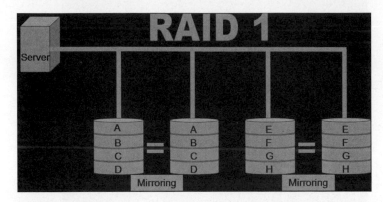

Figure 9-8 RAID 1.

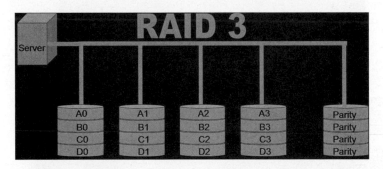

Figure 9-9 RAID 3.

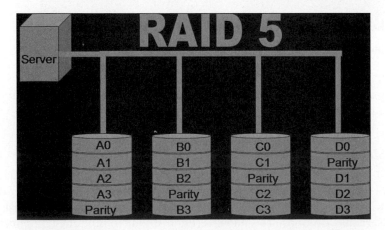

Figure 9-10 RAID 5.

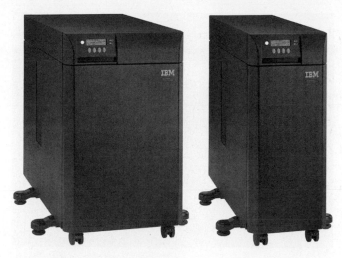

Figure 9-11 A DVD jukebox.
(Courtesy IBM.)

with the image manager to keep track of exactly where each image is located. The jukebox controller keeps like studies together as much as possible to minimize access time. The long-term archive has much higher access times than the short-term archive, but the price of storage per gigabyte is much less with the jukeboxes.

Optical Disk

Magneto-optical Disk
A **magneto-optical disk (MOD)** (Figure 9-12) is very similar to a compact disk (CD) or digital versatile disk (DVD) in that it is read optically with a laser, but the disk itself is housed within a plastic cartridge. MODs tend to be more reliable than some of the other long-term storage options. The disks are rather robust and can withstand many years of reading. They can be read faster than some of their counterparts. The cost per gigabyte is a bit higher for MODs than for some of the other long-term storage options, but it is still a viable long-term storage option.

Digital Versatile Disk
Digital versatile disks (DVDs) (Figure 9-13) were first introduced for use in video. CDs were used by a few early PACS adopters, but they found that the CDs could not hold enough data to make a CD archive cost and space efficient. DVDs have a much higher capacity. In 2006, a double-sided, two-layered DVD held 17 GB of data, whereas a CD held 650 MB. DVDs are the least expensive method for long-term archiving per gigabyte.

Ultra Density Optical
Ultra density optical (UDO) disk (Figure 9-14) is the new generation MOD. A UDO disk utilizes blue laser technology in its read and write activities. Plasmon (Plasmon PLC, Hertfordshire, UK) introduced the first UDO disk in 2004 with a disk

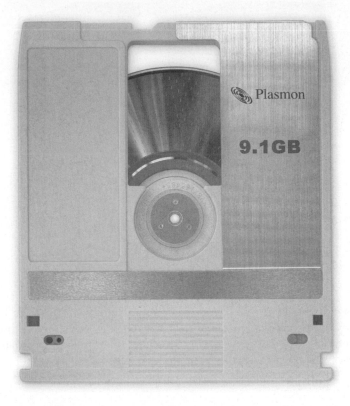

Figure 9-12 A magneto-optical disk (MOD).
(Courtesy Plasmon.)

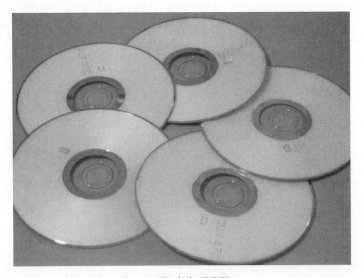

Figure 9-13 A digital versatile disk (DVD).

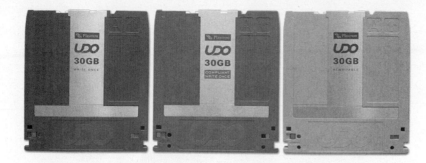

Figure 9-14 An ultra density optical (UDO) disk.
(Courtesy Plasmon.)

capacity of 30 GB (2006 MOD technology was at 9.1 GB), and the capacity is predicted to increase to 60 GB and then to 120 GB to accommodate industry needs. Currently, UDO technology operating costs are less than MODs and very competitive with DVD technology. The tape libraries being offered in 2006 held between 24 and 638 disks.

Tape

Tape (Figure 9-15) libraries provide the greatest scalability of the long-term archive options. These libraries can grow to hundreds of terabytes, possibly even a petabyte, and this technology will continue to improve and expand its storage limits. Tape is a fairly low-cost archive medium that comes in various sizes. These tapes are contained within a jukebox or library that has multiple drives and a robot arm to move the tapes in and out of the drives. These libraries can hold between 10 and 1448 tapes in one library (Figure 9-16). Most of the libraries are scalable, meaning that additional libraries can be added to the original.

One of the biggest disadvantages of tape is its unreliability over multiple uses. The tape can wear after several years of heavy use and may become damaged. Tape also has a longer access time than its optical counterparts. Tape has greatly improved over the past few years in its speed and reliability, and it will continue to be a factor in long-term PACS archiving systems.

There are several types of magnetic tape technologies available:

- Linear tape open (LTO): LTO technology was developed jointly by Hewlett Packard (Palo Alto, CA), IBM (Armonk, NY), and Quantum (San Jose, CA) to make available an open-format tape storage option. Open-format technology means that users have multiple sources of product and media that enable them to mix products from various vendors and still maintain compatibility and function.
- The LTO format is a high-capacity tape technology. Current LTO-3 technology holds 400 GB of uncompressed data on a single tape.
- Digital linear tape (DLT): DLT technology was invented by Digital Equipment Corporation in 1984. It was purchased by Quantum in 1994, and they license the technology. DLT tape drives have storage capacities between 40 and 160 GB, and a newer DLT technology known as super DLT has a capacity of 160 to 300 GB uncompressed.

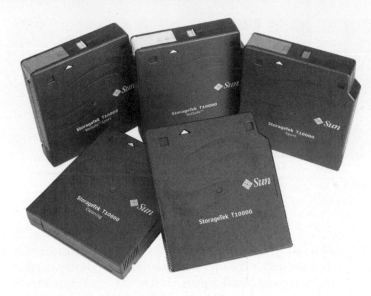

Figure 9-15 A magnetic tape.
(Courtesy Sun Microsystems.)

- Advanced intelligent tape (AIT): AIT is a high-speed and high-capacity tape made by Sony (Tokyo, Japan) to compete with the DLT. Sony introduced AIT in 1996 with a tape capacity of 25 GB; current AIT-4 technology has a capacity of 200 GB. Sony developed the next generation of AIT tapes, known as SAIT, and they have an initial capacity of 500 GB. Sony plans for the fourth generation of SAIT to come out by 2010 with a capacity of 4 TB/tape.

Magnetic Disk

As mentioned earlier in the chapter, as the price of **magnetic disk storage** (Figure 9-17) continues to decrease, RAID storage becomes a more feasible option for long-term storage. When using magnetic disks for long-term storage, the RAID arrays may be configured into three different but related fashions: direct attached storage (DAS), network attached storage (NAS), or storage area network (SAN).

- DAS (Figure 9-18): DAS is coupled to the system just like a short-term RAID. The DAS storage is connected directly via cable connections and shows up on the computer as different partitions for use. They are typically managed by the same RAID controller because in essence, the short-term RAID is just being expanded to have more storage space so that the studies will remain for a longer period of time.
- NAS (Figure 9-19): NAS servers are stand-alone RAID arrays that are attached directly to the network. Multiple NAS servers can be attached to one network to provide additional fault tolerance, and the load can be balanced throughout the servers.
- SAN (Figure 9-20): A SAN is a high-speed, special-purpose network (or subnetwork) that links different kinds of data storage devices with associated data servers,

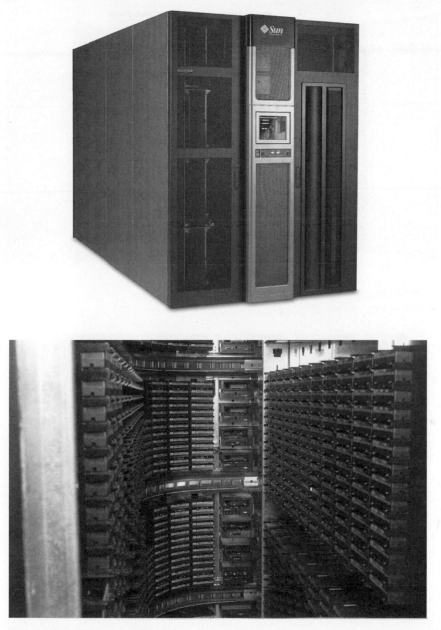

Figure 9-16 Various tape libraries.
(Courtesy Sun Microsystems.)

such as disk array controllers and tape libraries. SANs are becoming more popular in health care because of plummeting costs of magnetic disk storage. A SAN can be used by multiple departments within an institution and provide exceptional response speed for called-up data. The RAID levels can still be taken advantage of when they are used in conjunction with a SAN.

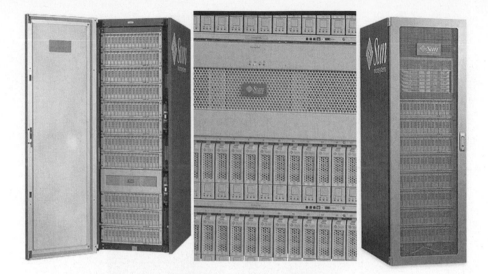

Figure 9-17 Magnetic disk storage used as a long-term archive.
(Courtesy Sun Microsystems.)

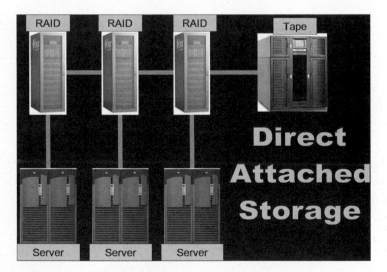

Figure 9-18 A direct attached storage long-term archive.

ARCHIVE CONSIDERATIONS

PACS archives are chosen for many reasons, including system need, system cost, and system compatibility. Many hospitals do not have the capital funds or the personnel to implement and operate the complex archive that is needed for a PACS. These hospitals have sought out other alternatives. One such alternative is an **application service provider (ASP).** An ASP is a company that provides outsourcing of archiving and

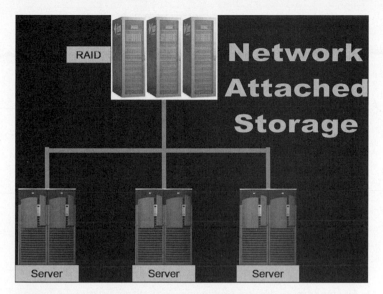

Figure 9-19 A network attached storage long-term archive.

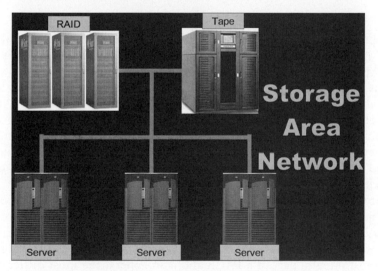

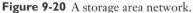

Figure 9-20 A storage area network.

management functions for a pay-per-use or pay-per-month charge. ASPs give smaller institutions access to the level of hardware and software they could not otherwise afford. Moreover, they assume responsibility for the day-to-day management of the archive system. Many ASP models have a short-term archive located on hospital premises, and the long-term archive is handled at the off-site location run by the ASP company (Figure 9-21). The short-term archive may be leased by the ASP, and the controller will prefetch images from the long-term off-site storage during the evening and night hours for the next day's schedule.

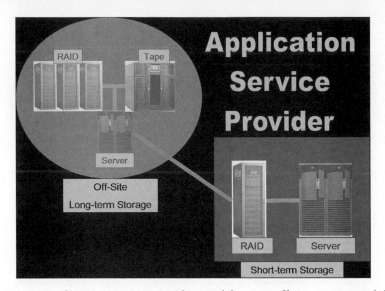

Figure 9-21 An application service provider model using off-site, outsourced long-term storage.

Another common use for an ASP is as a disaster recovery mechanism. **Disaster recovery** involves making copies of each tape or disk and sending them to another building or off-site location or by using the ASP model of shipping them to an outside company for storage on a pay-per-use policy. Even larger institutions have difficulty purchasing the proper amount of storage for disaster purposes. With proper disaster recovery, a complete copy of the archive is housed in another location and immediately available if the front-line archive goes down for any reason. With an ASP, however, the data may be housed in another state in a large storage silo, and the duplicated data may not be immediately available. There are many facets to disaster recovery, but a discussion of them is outside of the scope of this textbook. The most important thing to know is that backups are completed each day on the image manager database and that there must be some sort of contingency plan should disaster strike the archive room.

The archive is a complex arrangement of servers, databases, and storage devices. It is the most integral part of a PACS and is in general the most difficult piece to fully understand. This chapter presents an overview of the topic but by no means has presented the information needed to successfully purchase or operate a PACS archive.

SUMMARY

- The archive is a complex arrangement of computers and storage space that is the permanent location for digital images.
- The image manager contains the master database of everything that is in the archive.
- The archive server consists of the physical storage devices of the archive system.
- Most PACS archives are set up with short-term and long-term archive tiers.
- A short-term tier is commonly a RAID.
- A RAID is composed of several magnetic disks or hard drives that are linked together in an array.
- RAID 5 is the most common RAID level used in PACS archives.
- Long-term storage devices hold historic images for comparison reading on the workstations.
- Tape, optical disk, and magnetic disks are commonly used as long-term archive solutions.
- An ASP is a company that provides outsourcing of archiving and management functions for a pay-per-use or pay-per-month charge.
- A proper disaster recovery mechanism keeps a complete copy of the archive in another location that is immediately available in the event that the front line archive goes down.

CHAPTER REVIEW QUESTIONS

1. What is an image archive?

2. What are the two major categories of the image archive and describe their uses?

3. Define short-term archive, and give an example of the most common PACS short-term archive.

4. Define RAID, and describe the RAID levels addressed in the chapter.

5. Define long-term archive, and give several examples of those seen in a radiology department.

6. What is an ASP, and how can it be used in a radiology department?

CHAPTER 10

Digitizing, Printing, and Burning

1. Explain the differences between laser film digitizers and charge-coupled device (CCD) film digitizers.
2. Describe the uses of a film digitizer.
3. Compare and contrast dry laser imager technology with wet laser imager technology.
4. Discuss the common uses for imagers in a picture archival and communication system (PACS) environment.
5. Identify common uses for compact disk (CD)/ digital versatile disk (DVD) burners in a PACS environment.

KEY TERMS

Burner
Dry imager
Film digitizer

Teleradiology
Wet imager

PACS PERIPHERAL DEVICES

The previous chapters discussed the digital image acquisition process, picture archival and communication system (PACS) workstations, and archive systems. This chapter introduces you to three other components that are common in a PACS: film digitizers, imagers, and compact disk (CD) burners. Each of these three technologies plays an important role in the PACS.

FILM DIGITIZERS

Another way to take a projection radiograph to a digital format other than computed radiography (CR) and digital radiography (DR) is by using a film digitizer. The **film digitizer** (Figure 10-1) scans the analog film and produces numeric signals for each part of the scanned film. The numbers are fed into a software application that is

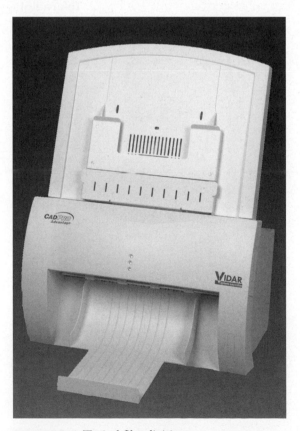

Figure 10-1 Typical film digitizer.
(Courtesy Vidar, Herndon, VA.)

attached to the scanner, and the scanner digitally reproduces the image using the numeric signals that represent each part of the radiograph.

There are two major types of film digitizers, one that uses laser technology and one that uses charge-coupled device (CCD) technology. Both are equal in quality, but currently the CCD digitizers are less expensive.

Laser Film Digitizers

A laser film digitizer uses a helium neon laser beam to convert the analog film image into a digital image (Figure 10-2). A laser inside the digitizer is bounced off a series of mirrors and scanned across the image. A photomultiplier tube picks up the light that is transmitted through the film. The laser scans one line at a time, and the photomultiplier picks up a very small area and then moves to the next area. The electrical signal is then sent to an analog-to-digital converter where the signal is translated into numbers based on the optical density of the film and the signal received. The numbers are then displayed on a monitor based on a look-up table (LUT) that indicates which shade of gray is associated with each number.

Laser digitizers are considered the gold standard for film digitization, and they have been around since approximately 1990. These digitizers can scan at various resolutions up to 5K and 12 bit, depending on the application need, and can scan an image in less than 25 seconds, depending on the scanning resolution. The disadvantages of laser digitizers include their expense and service needs, including maintenance, calibration, and quality control (QC) tests.

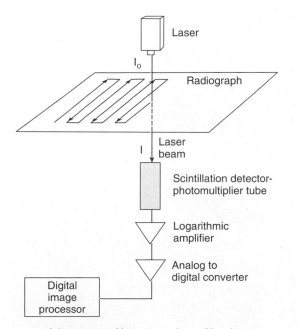

Figure 10-2 The process of digitizing a film using a laser film digitizer.

CCD Film Digitizers

A CCD film digitizer uses fluorescent bulbs that shine through the film and a CCD array that detects the light and transforms it into an electrical signal (Figure 10-3). The signal is then sent to an analog-to-digital converter and changed into a number that represents the intensity of light that passed through the film. As with the laser digitizer, the number is referenced against an LUT, and an image is displayed on a monitor.

The CCD digitizers are less expensive than the laser digitizers but somewhat slower. A CCD digitizer can take up to 80 seconds to scan one film through the digitizer, and it can also have problems with extreme light and dark areas on the film. However, the CCD digitizer image quality has improved over the years, and many radiologists say that the quality is adequate for their needs.

Common Uses of Digitizers

There are many uses for the film digitizer in the modern radiology department. Most departments list the following reasons for using a digitizer:

- **Teleradiology:** Teleradiology is a term used to describe the process of transferring digitized images for delivery at a distance to radiologists. Many hospitals use the digitizer to transfer films from off-site clinics to the main department for primary reading. The films are placed in the digitizer, and the image is transformed into a digital signal and sent via a network back to the main department. This saves the radiologist from having to drive to the remote location to read the few films that have been taken. It is also better patient care because films will be read much more quickly if sent digitally to the radiologist.
- Compare outside or old films: If a hospital has a PACS installed and is reporting the image from a monitor, it is very difficult to compare a film image with the

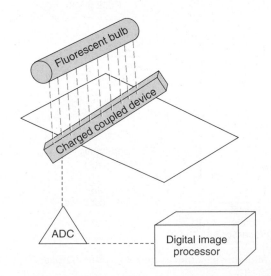

Figure 10-3 The process of digitizing a film using a CCD film digitizer.

image on the monitor. Many hospitals will digitize the patient's old films so that a comparison can be done much more easily. Patients also frequently come in with outside films. These are routinely digitized into the archive so that they can be referred to at a later date and compared with new digital images.

■ Film duplication: On occasion it is necessary to make duplicate copies of films. The film can be sent through the digitizer, and then the image can be printed onto film using a laser film imager.

■ Computed aided diagnosis (CAD): A new technology that is gaining momentum is CAD. It is most currently used in mammography and chest imaging. The film is sent through the digitizer, and a computer will analyze the densities seen on the image and alert the radiologist of questionable densities.

IMAGERS

Imagers, also known as film printers, receive an image from a workstation and print the image based on printer LUTs and preset print layouts. Both of these parameters vary for each modality that produces digital images. There are two major types of imagers that are still in use today: wet (chemical) laser imagers (Figure 10-4) and dry laser imagers (Figure 10-5).

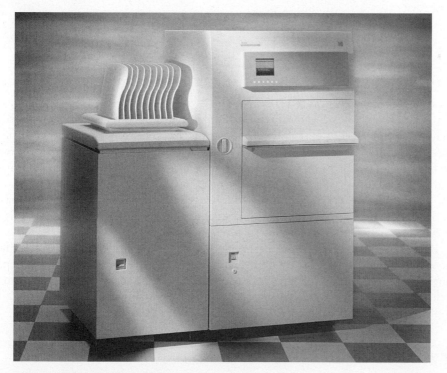

Figure 10-4 A wet laser imager.
(Courtesy Eastman Kodak Co., Rochester, NY.)

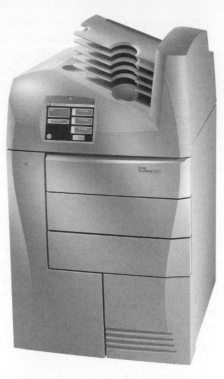

Figure 10-5 A dry laser imager.
(Courtesy Eastman Kodak Co., Rochester, NY.)

Wet Imagers

Wet imagers use chemicals to process the film that has been exposed to the laser. The laser beam produces an intensity of light that is proportional to the signal being received to regulate the optical density recorded on the film. The laser emits a red light, so the film that is used must be red sensitive. As mentioned earlier, conventional film has silver halide crystals suspended in an emulsion; the wet laser film is not much different other than being red sensitive so that the laser may etch the image into the film. Because this film is sensitive to red light, it must be placed in its film magazine and processed in total darkness. This processing takes place in a bath of chemicals just like film used in the traditional film/screen department.

Because wet imagers require chemicals, they must be placed in a well-ventilated area with proper drainage and plumbing. Because of these requirements, fewer departments install this type of imager. Wet imagers also take up much more space than the dry imagers, and the cost of chemicals, disposal, and maintenance make them a less popular choice than dry imagers.

Dry Imagers

Dry imagers use heat to process the latent image that is etched into the silver emulsion by the laser. Just like conventional film, dry laser film also has silver within its emulsion, but instead of silver halide crystals, the dry film has silver behenate. The film is exposed with a laser in a fashion similar to the wet imager. The silver salts are then exposed to heat and turn to metallic silver to create the image on the film.

Dry imagers have been found to have slightly worse quality than wet imagers, but the dry imagers take up less space and require no special locations. The dry imager film quality tends to degrade over time, and it is more sensitive to heat and humidity than conventional film, especially if the film is stored in a warm environment. Moreover, because the chemicals that make the image are still on the film after it is processed, the image can gain more density when stored in a high heat area. The major advantage to the dry imager is that it only requires an outlet and a network connection to connect to the departmental modalities.

Common Uses of Imagers

Even though the future of radiology is a filmless environment, there will always be a need for producing a hardcopy film. The following paragraphs outline a few reasons why film can and will be used in the "filmless" radiology department.

- Backup: The ability to print just in case the PACS goes down is one of the most often heard explanations. In most hospital networks, the modalities are set up to send not only to the PACS but also directly to a laser imager. So if the PACS is down for some reason, the modality can still print directly to the imager.
- Difficult PACS locations: When a PACS is installed, there are a few departments that are difficult to convert to PACS initially, like surgery, orthopedics, and sometimes the emergency room. In surgery, space is at a premium, and it may be difficult to place a PACS workstation in the surgical suite. In many instances, films are printed for surgery and placed on a lightbox.
- Outside physicians: Many referring physicians prefer to see their patient's images while reviewing the radiologist's report. When installing a PACS, one of the last pieces to be converted is outside physician access so, with imagers, films can be printed and sent to the physicians as normal.
- Legal cases: For legal cases, films can be printed to be viewed in court. It may become more commonplace to have computer access in the courtroom, and at that time images can be viewed digitally.
- Teaching purposes: Most hospitals train students at their institution. The printing of films for training purposes will continue to be a need.

CD/DVD BURNERS

Early PACS advocates used cost savings to justify purchasing a PACS, but you have seen that there remains a need for hard copies. Film printing is a costly part of a PACS because laser film is expensive, more expensive than conventional film. Most hospitals try to reduce the amount of printing done in the department. One alternative to printing hard copies is to burn images to an optical disk.

Remember from Chapter 2 that CDs and digital versatile disks (DVDs) are both thin injection-molded polycarbonate plastic disks. The disk is impressed from a mold to form microscopic bumps that indicate either a 1 or 0 to the computer. Over the bumps is a reflective layer of aluminum covered with a clear protective coat of acrylic. In a DVD there are multiple layers of the polycarbonate plastic. Aluminum is used behind the inner layers, and gold is used behind the outer layers. The gold is semireflective so the laser can penetrate to the inner layers of plastic. With a **burner,** the information is burned onto the disk starting in the center and spiraling out to the edge of the disk. The laser will burn a tiny depression (pit) into the disk to represent the data being saved. A burned disk will be a series of pits and lands, areas that were not burned by the laser (Figure 10-6).

All PACS vendors offer the ability to burn images to a CD or DVD for purpose of sharing the images outside of the PACS. When a disk is burned with the patient's images, a digital imaging and communications in medicine (DICOM) viewer is also burned onto the disk. When the disk is put into a drive, the software automatically launches and displays the images. The software is generally very intuitive and easy to use and allows for minor image enhancements such as window/level adjustments and simple measurements.

Common Uses of Burners

These disks can be used in most of the same applications as the printed film with the exception of using them as a fail-safe mechanism and for those departments that are in difficult locations. Many referring physicians prefer having the images on disk rather than film because it takes up less space, can be added directly to the patient's office chart, and the images can be manipulated.

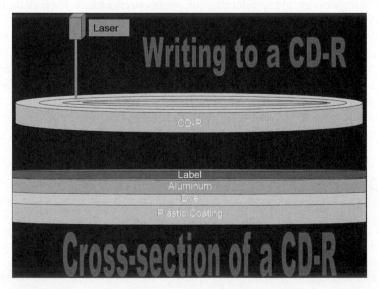

Figure 10-6 The process of burning an image to a CD.

Disks also are much cheaper to produce and send out to physicians. One sheet of dry laser film is approximately $0.48, whereas a CD is approximately $0.28. The CD can hold multiple studies, and multiple sheets of film would be needed to print an entire study. The CD will also be much cheaper to mail than the film. Disks will become much more common outside of the radiology department as the advantages are seen by those outside of the department.

SUMMARY

- A film digitizer scans the analog film and produces numeric signals for each part of the scanned film.
- A laser film digitizer uses a helium neon laser beam to convert the analog film image into a digital image.
- A CCD film digitizer uses fluorescent bulbs that shine through the film and a CCD array that detects the light and transforms the light into an electrical signal.
- Imagers, also known as film printers, receive an image from a workstation and print the image based on printer LUTs and preset print layouts.
- Dry imagers use heat to process the latent image that is etched into the silver emulsion by the laser.
- Wet imagers use chemicals to process the film that has been exposed to the laser.
- A CD/DVD burner can burn images to be shared outside of the radiology department. Along with the images, a DICOM viewer is burned to the disk for ease of viewing.

CHAPTER REVIEW QUESTIONS

1. How does a laser digitizer digitize a film?

2. How does a CCD digitizer digitize a film?

3. What are the common uses of a digitizer?

4. What is a wet laser imager, and how does it work?

5. What is a dry laser imager, and how does it work?

6. What are the common uses of film imagers?

7. How are CD/DVD burners used in a radiology department?

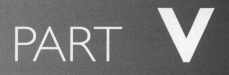

PART V

Quality Control and Quality Management

CHAPTER 11

Ensuring Quality in PACS

1. Describe the differences between quality control (QC) and quality assurance activities.
2. Define continuous quality improvement and its uses in a radiology department.
3. Describe the daily and monthly/quarterly monitor QC activities.
4. Discuss the process of daily/weekly QC on laser imagers.
5. State the common QC activities used to measure system speed and data integrity.
6. Describe several quality assurance activities used in a digital radiology department.

KEY TERMS

Acceptance testing
Continuous quality improvement
Error maintenance
PACS administrator
Photometer

Quality assurance
Quality control
Routine maintenance
Super user
The Joint Commission

QUALITY ASPECTS

When you think of quality, what is the first thing that comes to mind? Is it the service at a restaurant or the backpack purchased at the beginning of the semester? Both of these deal with quality in some way: one is people-centered, and the other is product-centered. Likewise, radiology has both a people-centered quality and a product-centered quality.

The traditional department with film and chemistry has many quality procedures that must be followed. Many of these same protocols are used in the digital department, but they have been modified to be relevant to digital equipment and processes.

The next section introduces the terms used to talk about quality within a radiology department. The following sections introduce various routines that should be done in the department to ensure that the picture archival and communication system (PACS) is functioning properly and that the images are being produced at a certain quality level. Chapter 12 discusses quality with cassette-based and cassette-less digital radiographic equipment and processes.

TERMS OF QUALITY

Quality has always been a part of health care, whether as a service or product. Health care institutions pride themselves on providing the highest quality possible, and they put many measures into place to ensure that the highest quality is provided to each patient. The ultimate focus in health care is to improve patient care and provide a high quality service so that patients will want to return. Most health care institutions are accredited by **the Joint Commission** (TJC), formerly know as the Joint Commission on the Accreditation of Healthcare Organizations (JCAHO). This accreditation is voluntary but necessary in many instances to obtain Medicaid certification, hold certain licenses, obtain reimbursements from insurance companies, and receive malpractice insurance. Today TJC uses a more all encompassing term of continuous quality improvement (CQI) or total quality management (TQM). The next few sections will define these concepts and provide some basic applications in a digital department.

Quality Assurance

Quality assurance (QA) can be defined as a plan for the systematic observation and assessment of the different aspects of a project, service, or facility to make certain that standards of quality are being met. QA activities are focused around people and service. In a radiology department there are many processes involved in the day-to-day activities. For example, once a patient has been checked-in at the front desk, there is a process that is followed to alert the technologist that a patient is waiting. If this process is not followed, the patient may have to wait for an extended period before a technologist arrives to check for waiting patients. This extended wait time affects patient care in a negative manner, and therefore it will be seen as poor quality of service. A QA measure should be in place to monitor patient wait times to ensure that the process of alerting a technologist that a patient is waiting is working properly.

Most QA activities will produce quantitative data that can be analyzed. These data can be used to monitor the processes and determine whether the process is working as it should and whether the standard of quality has been met.

Quality Control

Quality control (QC) can be defined as a comprehensive set of activities designed to monitor and maintain systems that produce a product. QC measures are taken to ensure that radiologic procedures are performed safely, are appropriate for the patient, are performed efficiently, and produce a high-quality image. For example, tests are performed on the radiographic room to make sure that all of the parts are functioning properly, such as the collimator, generator, and focal spots. All of these parts make up the whole of the room, and if one part is off, it can cause harm to the patient or reduce the quality of the examination.

QC measures are required by law to maintain the license for the room or department. The data from the various activities are kept by a designated individual within the department. Most QC activities are part of a QA program, and the data are used to improve the quality of the processes and department. There are three major categories of QC test that are used at various times:

- **Acceptance testing:** This type of testing is performed before newly installed or majorly repaired equipment can be accepted by the department. The testing may be performed by a designated technologist, a radiation physicist, or by service personnel employed by the hospital. The acceptance testing is used to determine whether the equipment is performing within the vendor's specifications and as promised.
- **Routine maintenance:** Routine maintenance is performed to ensure that the equipment is performing as expected. This type of testing can catch problems before they become radiographically apparent. This testing may be performed by a designated technologist, a radiation physicist, or by service personnel employed by the vendor.
- **Error maintenance:** When errors occur in equipment performance, corrective action must occur. Errors will be detected by poor equipment performance or poor quality outcomes. These corrections will generally be done by service personnel employed by the vendor.

Continuous Quality Improvement

Continuous quality improvement (CQI) tends to focus on the process rather than on the people or the service. The belief is that if the process is good, health care workers will follow it, and service will be good. The CQI process does not replace QA/QC programs. The QA/QC programs focus on maintaining a certain level of quality, not necessarily improving to a higher quality. CQI focuses on improving the process or system within which the people function as team members rather than focus on an individual's work.

One of the most important concepts to understand with CQI is that all levels of people within the organization must be involved in the process of improvement.

Because CQI focuses not on individuals and their mistakes but rather on the process, each team member is more apt to participate in improving the organization. It is very important that everyone participate because if one spoke is not involved, the wheel will fall off, and the quality cart cannot move forward.

PACS EQUIPMENT QC

When beginning a QC program, care must be taken to document all surrounding variables so that each quality measure can be repeated without harm to the process. Documentation is very important in any QC activity, and it must be kept up to date to make a valid performance measure. As with all quality activities, documentation is the most difficult part of the process and the easiest part to not complete. Without the documentation to back up the findings, it will be difficult to prove the need for repair or update of a system.

The next several sections focus on QC activities that should be monitored in a PACS environment, including display quality for both monitor and film, processing speed, network transfer speed, and the data integrity of data that are called back from the archive. This is not an all-encompassing list. Many vendors have suggestions for what should be monitored for their systems. It is very important that you follow the vendor's list and timetable for these various activities. According to the American College of Radiology (ACR) "Technical Standard for Digital Image Data Management":

> Any facility using a digital image data management system must have documented policies and procedures for monitoring and evaluating the effective management, safety, and proper performance of acquisition, digitization, compression, transmission, display, archiving, and retrieval functions of the system. The quality control program should be designed to maximize the quality and accessibility of diagnostic information.

The ACR also suggests that all the quality tests described below be carried out with a Society of Motion Pictures and Television Engineers (SMPTE) test pattern (Figure 11-1) to ensure continuity of measurements. A test pattern developed by the American Association of Physicists in Medicine (AAPM) Task Group 18 (TG18) (Figure 11-2) is also becoming more widely accepted for use in these QC tests. The ACR suggests that QC tasks be performed at least monthly, whereas the AAPM has a much more rigorous schedule. The AAPM suggests that the testing be performed on acceptance and annually by a trained physicist, and the daily and monthly/quarterly tests can be performed by a trained QC technologist or a physicist. If any of the following tests fails or produces out-of-range readings, corrective action and continued monitoring should be done. Follow your department's policy on equipment maintenance procedures. It may be necessary to contact your radiation physicist to follow up on your findings.

Monitor Quality

The monitor is often the weakest link in the digital imaging chain. The monitor has a direct effect on the quality of the image that is presented to the radiologist for reading or to the referring physician for review. Unfortunately, it is not cost-effective to provide the highest quality monitor for all viewing situations. As discussed in Chapter 8,

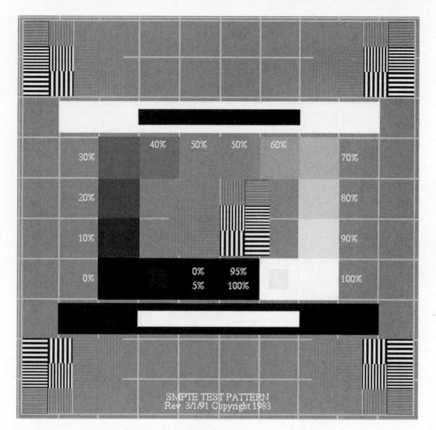

Figure 11-1 SMPTE test pattern.

the radiologist workstation will have the highest quality medical grade monitors, usually 2K or 3K for computed radiography (CR) or digital radiography (DR), 1K or 2K for cross-sectional images, and up to 4K for mammography. As with digital cameras, the megapixel measurement may also be used to determine the appropriate monitor. Generally, the physician review workstations and the technologist QC workstations have high quality commercial monitors. They usually have a resolution of 1K.

The following QC recommendations for display monitors come from the AAPM in their document entitled "Assessment for Display Performance for Medical Imaging Systems." This document outlines testing to be completed both by physicists and by technologists/users. The following paragraphs outline the tasks to be completed by a trained technologist on a daily and monthly/quarterly basis on all monitors used to view images.

Daily Monitor QC

- Turn on the monitor, and allow it ample time to warm up.
- Make sure that the monitor is dust-free on the viewing surface and near the airflow areas.

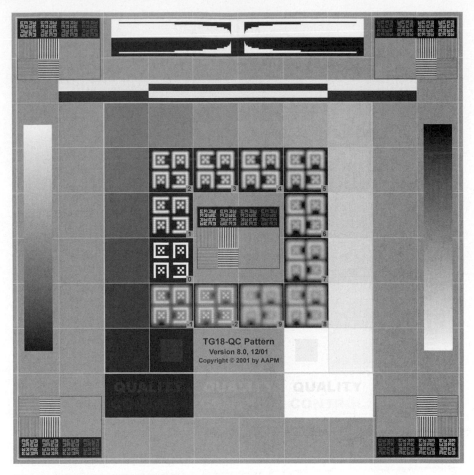

Figure II-2 AAPM TG18-QC test pattern.

- Retrieve a QC monitor test pattern (SMPTE or AAPM TG18-QC). (The retrieval time may also be noted for a later test to be discussed.)
- General image quality and appearance: Evaluate the overall appearance of the pattern, and take note of any nonuniformities or artifacts, especially at black-to-white and white-to-black transitions. Verify that the vertical and horizontal bars appear continuous.
- Geometric distortion: Make sure that the borders and lines of the pattern are clear and straight and that the pattern appears to be centered in the active area of the display.
- Luminance, reflection, noise, and glare: Verify that all 16 luminance patches are clearly visible. If desired, measure their luminance using a luminance meter or **photometer,** a device used to measure the luminescence of areas on the monitor (Figure 11-3). Evaluate the results in comparison to previous measurements. Make sure that the 5% and 95% patches are clearly visible, and evaluate the appearance

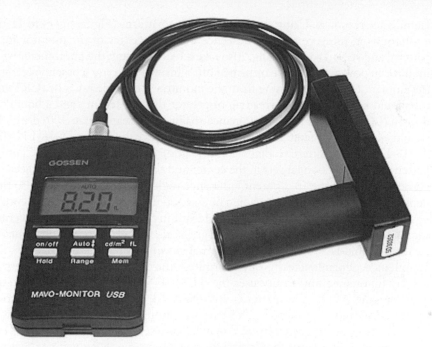

Figure 11-3 A photometer used to measure luminescence.

of low-contrast letters and the targets at the corners of all luminance patches with and without ambient lighting.

■ Resolution: Evaluate the Cx patterns at the center and corners of the pattern, and verify that all letters and numbers appear.

Monthly/Quarterly Monitor QC

■ Turn on the monitor, and allow it ample time to warm up.

■ Make sure that the monitor is dust-free on the viewing surface and near the air-flow areas.

■ Retrieve a QC monitor test pattern.

■ Geometric distortions: Using the TG18-QC test pattern, maximize it to fill the entire usable display area. For rectangular display areas, the patterns should cover at least the narrower aspect of the display area and be placed at the center of the area used for image viewing. The pattern should be examined from a normal viewing distance, and the linearity of the pattern should be checked visually across the display area and at the edges.

■ Reflection: Determine whether there are other light sources like overhead lights, other monitors, or viewboxes that are reflecting back off of the monitor. Eliminate or reduce these sources of light if possible, and view test pattern at a normal viewing distance.

- Luminance response: Using the TG18-LN test patterns (Figures 11-4 to 11-6) and a photometer, measure the luminescence from the center of the monitor for each pattern, and record each reading. Also take a reading using the photometer with the monitor in power-save mode or turned off. This will give you a baseline reading for the ambient luminance coming from the monitor. A cathode ray tube (CRT) monitor should have a luminance reading of greater than $170\,cd/m^2$, and a liquid crystal display (LCD) should have a luminance reading of greater than $100\,cd/m^2$. There should also be a greater than $250\,cd/m^2$ difference between TG18-LN-01 and TG18-LN-18 test pattern readings (contrast ratio). Using the TG18-CT (Figure 11-7) pattern, the half-moon targets in the center and the four low-contrast objects at the corners of each of the 16 different luminance regions should be visible. Also the bit-depth resolution of the display should be assessed using the TG18-MP (Figure 11-8) test pattern. The assessment includes determining whether the horizontal contouring bands, their relative locations, and grayscale reversals are within limits. Both patterns should be examined from a normal viewing distance.
- Luminance dependencies: Nonuniformity—the visual method for determining display luminance uniformity uses the TG18-UN10 and TG18-UN80 test patterns (Figure 11-9). The patterns are displayed, and the uniformity across the displayed pattern is assessed. The patterns should be observed from a normal viewing distance. Angular response may be assessed visually using the TG18-CT test pattern. The pattern should first be viewed on-axis to determine the visibility of all half-moon targets. The viewing angle at which any of the contrast thresholds

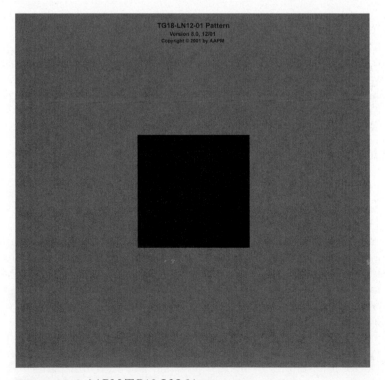

Figure 11-4 AAPM TG18-LN-01 test pattern.

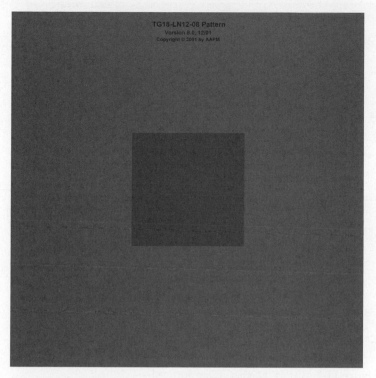

Figure 11-5 AAPM TG18-LN-08 test pattern.

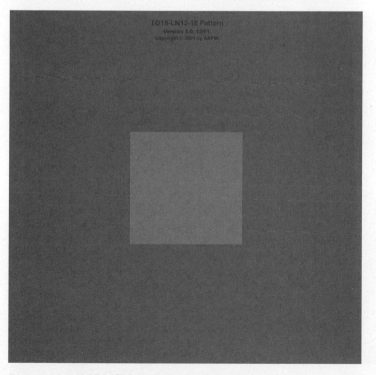

Figure 11-6 AAPM TG18-LN-18 test pattern.

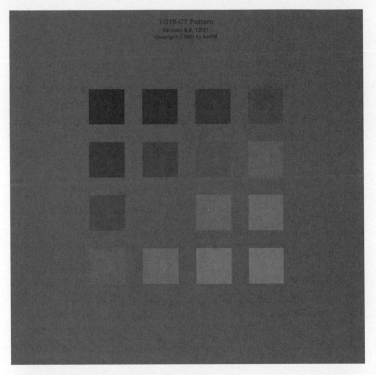

Figure 11-7 AAPM TG18-CT test pattern.

Figure 11-8 AAPM TG18-MP test pattern.

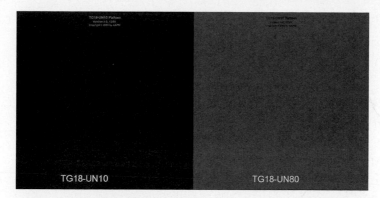

Figure 11-9 AAPM TG18-UN10 and TG18-UN80 test patterns.

become invisible should be noted. Using the TG18-UNL10 and TG18-UNL80 test patterns (Figure 11-10), luminance is measured at five positions over the monitor (center and four corners) using a calibrated photometer. The five readings should be within 30% of one another.

■ Resolution: Using the TG18-QC pattern and the magnifying glass within the PACS software, examine the displayed Cx patterns at the center and four corners of the monitor. The line pair patterns in the horizontal and vertical directions should also be evaluated in terms of visibility, and the average brightness of the patterns should also be assessed using the grayscale step pattern as a reference. Note any difference in appearance of the test patterns between the horizontal and vertical lines. The relative width of the black and white lines in these patches should also be examined using the magnifying glass. The resolution uniformity may be determined by using the TG18-CX (Figure 11-11) test pattern and magnifying glass in the same way that the Cx elements in the TG18-QC pattern were used.

As mentioned earlier, all annual testing and acceptance testing should be performed by a qualified medical physicist. They follow their own standard set of tests to make sure that the monitors are performing up to their capabilities.

Printer Image Quality

Besides the PACS, the printed image is another way to distribute images around the hospital enterprise. As with monitors, there are several steps that should be taken to ensure that the image being seen is of consistent quality.

Wet Laser Imager
Daily/Weekly QC

■ Monitor each film printed to ensure that it is free from artifacts and that it matches monitor or desired quality.

■ Print a test pattern from the PACS. Some printers have a built-in test pattern that can be printed by depressing a button on the printer.

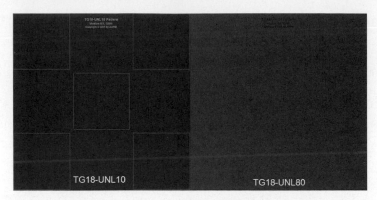

Figure 11-10 AAPM TG18-UNL10 and TG18-UNL80 test patterns.

■ Observe the printed test pattern for artifacts and changes in density, contrast, and resolution.

■ Measure the steps on the test pattern using a densitometer, and document your findings. Create a characteristic curve to compare previous measurements.

■ Monitor the processing mechanism as you would any chemical processor. Note the temperature, as well as the fixer, developer, and wash levels. Clean the racks and rollers as appropriate.

■ Make sure that the preventative maintenance schedule is completed in a timely manner, and maintain documentation of the completion and findings.

Dry Laser Imager

Daily/Weekly QC

■ Monitor each film printed to ensure that it is free from artifacts and that it matches monitor or desired quality.

■ Print a test pattern from the PACS. Some printers have a built-in test pattern that can be printed by depressing a button on the printer.

■ Observe the printed test pattern for artifacts and changes in density, contrast, and resolution.

■ Measure the steps on the test pattern using a densitometer, and document your findings. Create a characteristic curve to compare previous measurements.

■ Make sure that the preventative maintenance schedule is completed in a timely manner, and maintain documentation of the completion and findings.

Speed

Speed is always a concern in the radiology department, whether it is the speed at which patients are brought back for their x-rays or the speed at which the radiologist gets a final report signed. It is no different in a digital department, but there are other considerations when talking about speed: the processing speed of the workstation and the image retrieval/transfer rate.

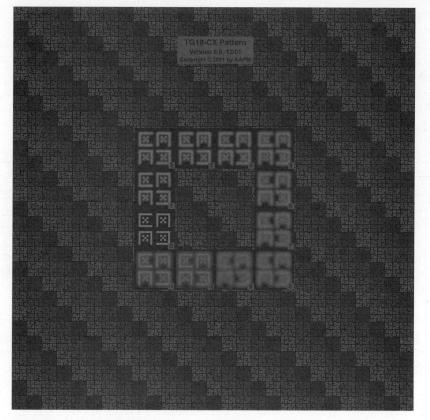

Figure 11-11 AAPM TG18-CX test pattern.

Workstation Processing Speed

The workstation processing speed can be measured or documented in many different ways. The following is a practical way to monitor the speed of your workstation.

- Determine a study to be used as your test. You must use the same study each time to ensure there are no variables. Choose a study with several images and a patient that has several studies.
- Open the initial test study, and note the loading speed. Page through the images, and note the loading speed of each image.
- Choose an image processing function appropriate for the test images that you have chosen, such as edge enhancement, stitching, or a three-dimensional (3D) processing function. Perform the function, and note the processing speed. Use the same tool each time you perform the test to maintain consistency.
- Open the patient's next study using the appropriate PACS function. Note the loading speed of the images.

After acceptance of the workstation, this procedure should be followed weekly to establish a pattern. If no changes are seen, this procedure can then be done on a monthly basis. Anytime the software or equipment is updated, the procedure should be done on a weekly basis until a pattern is established again.

Image Transfer Speed

Image transfer speed should be monitored from the modality to PACS and from the archive to a workstation. The following steps are an easy way to monitor these transfer speeds:

- Determine a study to be used as your test. You must use the same study each time to ensure there are no variables. You can also use test patterns that you have saved on your archive. The procedure should be done on the same day of the week and at approximately the same time to reduce network traffic variables.
- Retrieve the study to the workstation. Note the amount of time it took the entire study to arrive at the workstation.
- To test the transfer speed from the modalities, have each modality send their QC images to the archive, and note the amount of time the transfer takes. Make sure that the modality sends the exact same image set each time you test.

After acceptance of the system, this procedure should be followed weekly to establish a pattern. If no changes are seen, this procedure can then be done on a monthly basis. Anytime the software or equipment is updated, the procedure should be done on a weekly basis until a pattern is established again.

Data QC

Data Integrity

A constant measure to be monitored is whether all images completed at the modality make it to the PACS. This is usually caught by the radiologist, but as a technologist, it is a good practice to monitor this periodically. After initial installation, you should check on a daily basis to make sure that all of the images that you sent to the PACS arrived on the PACS. If there are no missing images for several weeks, this practice can be scaled back to once a week. You can randomly choose several studies that were sent during the week to determine whether all of the images made it to the PACS.

Another test for data integrity is to periodically pull up images from the archive to make sure the same images sent initially are still in the study after archival. This should also be done on a weekly basis.

After acceptance of the system, this procedure should be followed daily to establish a pattern. If no changes are seen, this procedure can then be done weekly and then on a monthly basis. Anytime the software or equipment is updated, the procedure should be done on a daily basis until a pattern is established again.

Compression Recall

Compression is used to reduce the size of the image files to increase the speed of the network transfer of the images. Compression protocols need to be established by your radiologists and radiation physicist. They will determine the level of compression that will be acceptable for your institution. The following steps are a practical way of observing compression recall of images:

- Save several versions of the AAPM TG18-QC test pattern on your archive using different compression ratios as follows:
  - No compression
  - Lossless compression (2:1 compression ratio)
  - Lossy compression (variable compression ratios—use the ratio that your department uses, if any)
- Recall all test patterns, and compare the results of no compression, lossless, and lossy. Determine whether there is any loss of information on the compressed images. Note any changes in image quality, if any.

PACS CQI

There are many processes used each day in a PACS environment, and each of these processes should be monitored to make sure that the PACS is functioning up to its capabilities. Remember that CQI activities revolve around process rather than people and systems. The next few sections describe several simple CQI activities that need to be monitored in a radiology department. Many activities that are monitored before the digital conversion of the department should continue after the conversion. Each PACS vendor may have different activities that they recommend. All of these activities should be adhered to so that your PACS will run up to its potential, and problems can be found before they cause major system downtime.

Recognition of Undiagnostic Images

One CQI activity that should be monitored is the documentation of undiagnostic images being forwarded to the PACS. This activity will be primarily carried out by the radiologists. If a poor quality image is detected by the radiologist, the study and performing technologist are noted, and the information is shared with the lead technologist or the PACS administrator to follow up with the performing technologist.

The radiologist may note the areas and reasons for the poor quality image. If the poor quality image was caused by equipment malfunction, the appropriate QC test should be carried out, and the appropriate service protocol followed. If the poor quality image was operator error, additional training or counseling by the supervisor may be required.

System Up-Time

Another common QA activity is the monitoring of how often the system is down for any reason. A log should be kept to note any time that the system is down. Also in the log note the reason, how long, what had to be done to fix the problem, and who fixed the problem. If the same problem continues to occur, this log can be used to prove that either a piece of equipment needs to be replaced or that additional service is needed.

System Training

System training is a very important activity that must never stop. One of the early misconceptions of installing a PACS is that the vendor applications training would be sufficient for training all staff that interact with the PACS. This is far from the truth. The vendor applications personnel are usually on site for 1 to 2 weeks during initial installation. The vendor applications training is supposed to train several **super users** (people who are trained on all aspects of the system and are prepared to train others) and help set up the system to site specifications.

The super users and the **PACS administrator** (the person trained to oversee the PACS) need to set up an ongoing training program. The training program must include several skill levels, from the radiologist to the technologist to the ancillary personnel. Each new employee needs to be trained on the system. Each time that a new version of the software is installed, the training protocol needs to be revised; retraining of existing personnel may be necessary. Each department also has a list of skills that are tested and retrained each year. PACS skills should be included in this annual training. A training record should be kept for each employee to show proof of skills.

SUMMARY

- Most hospitals are voluntarily accredited by TJC. This accreditation is necessary to obtain Medicaid certification, hold certain licenses, obtain reimbursements from insurance companies, and receive malpractice insurance.
- QA can be defined as a plan for the systematic observation and assessment of the different aspects of a project, service, or facility to make certain that standards of quality are being met.
- QC can be defined as a comprehensive set of activities designed to monitor and maintain systems that produce a product.
- Acceptance testing is performed before newly installed or substantially repaired equipment being accepted by the department.
- Routine maintenance is performed to ensure that the equipment is performing as expected.
- Error maintenance occurs when errors are detected in equipment performance.
- CQI tends to focus on the process rather than the people or the service. CQI focuses on improving the process or system in which people function as members of a team rather than focus on the individual's work.
- The following QC activities should take place on a prescribed basis:
  - Daily and monthly/quarterly monitor QC
  - Printer image quality
  - Speed assessment
  - Data QC
- Most CQI activities that were in place before the conversion to a digital department should continue. Others should be developed, such as system up-time and system training.

CHAPTER REVIEW QUESTIONS

1. What are the differences between quality control and quality assurance activities?

2. What is the definition of continuous quality improvement, and what are its uses in the radiology department?

3. What are the quality control activities that should be performed on the computer monitors in the radiology department, and how often should these activities be performed?

4. What are the quality control activities that should be performed on the laser imagers in the radiology department, and how often should these activities be performed?

5. How would system speed and data integrity be measured as part of the QC program?

6. Describe several quality assurance activities used in a digital radiology department.

CHAPTER 12

Total Quality Management of CR and DR Systems

Total Quality Management

Quality Control Standards

Quality Control Schedules and Responsibilities

1. Discuss total quality management (QM) and its uses in digital imaging.
2. Describe the daily, weekly, and monthly quality control (QC) activities assigned to a radiologic technologist.
3. Explain the importance of establishing a repeat analysis database with digital imaging.
4. State the common QC activities performed by a service engineer on digital radiographic equipment.
5. Become familiar with problem-reporting responsibilities.
6. Recognize the QM/QC activities to be performed by the radiation physicist.
7. Acknowledge personal responsibilities for correctly marking images, maintaining personal repeat rates, and preventing artifacts.

KEY TERMS

Continuous quality improvement (CQI)
Preventative maintenance (PM)

Quality control (QC)
Total quality management (TQM)

TOTAL QUALITY MANAGEMENT

Quality control (QC) standards for image acquisition, processing, and equipment maintenance all contribute to the concept of **total quality management (TQM)** or **continuous quality improvement (CQI),** as discussed in Chapter 11. The overall efficiency and effectiveness of imaging systems are evaluated beyond the mechanics of producing radiographic images. This chapter introduces the concept of whole system evaluation, considering image acquisition, processing, and evaluation, as well as repeat examination analysis, communication issues, and system problem identification.

QUALITY CONTROL STANDARDS

The American College of Radiology requires compliance with standards of practice to ensure quality in any imaging system. Three general areas define digital image quality: contrast, resolution, and noise. These must be monitored to avoid unnecessary repeat examinations and overexposure to patients and staff. There are a number of system tests that must be performed by service personnel and/or radiologic technologists and radiation physicists. With the increased sophistication of digital radiographic equipment, it is critical that these tests be performed in a consistent and thorough manner. The following sections are in no way an exhaustive list of activities that should be performed. The manufacturer's suggested list of systems tests should be performed as outlined in the equipment and service manuals.

The American Association of Physicists in Medicine is another organization instrumental in publishing standard quality control activities for the radiologic sciences. It first formed a task group to address acceptance testing and quality control of photostimulable storage phosphor imaging systems or computed radiography. It published the AAPM Report No. 93. This report outlines generic QC tests performed by diagnostic radiologic physicists and radiologic technologists. The report also documents an overview of basic CR systems, typical specifications, and testing procedures. The student is highly encouraged to retrieve this report posted at www.aapm.org. The report's ISBN is 9781888340648 and the title is "Acceptance Testing and Quality Control of Photostimulable Storage Phosphor Imaging Systems." The AAPM is also working on a report entitled "Acceptance Testing and Quality Control of Digital Radiographic Imaging Systems." This report is not expected until sometime in 2011. Again, please refer to the manufacturer's equipment manual for suggested system QC tests for all digital equipment.

QUALITY CONTROL SCHEDULES AND RESPONSIBILITIES

The radiologic technologist is the first line of defense in preventing, recognizing, and reporting QC issues. **Quality control (QC)** is defined as a comprehensive set of activities designed to monitor and maintain a system or piece of equipment. The complicated and delicate nature of digital equipment necessitates frequent and consistent oversight to avoid image errors and unnecessary patient exposure. The following is a schedule for proper computed radiology (CR)/digital radiology (DR) system maintenance.

Technologist Responsibilities

Daily (Box 12-1)

- General system inspection, including:
  - Cleanliness of cassettes
    - Are the cassettes free of dirt and debris on all surfaces? Dirt on the cassette may obscure the laser reader photomultiplier, leaving artifacts or reader errors.
    - Are barcode labels in good condition and able to be read? Labels in disrepair will compromise the connection of the imaging plate identification to the patient and examination identification information.
  - Hinge and latch inspection
    - Are hinges and/or latches in good condition? Broken latches or hinges can damage readers and will require a service call to get the reader in working order.
  - Erasure of imaging plates
    - Have plates been left unexposed for longer than 24 hours? Even cassettes that have been erased more recently have the potential to record exposure such as prolonged light exposure or scatter radiation. The safest procedure is to erase cassettes before use if unsure of the last erasure performed.
  - Verification of digital interfaces and network transmission
    - Is the reader communicating with the workstation? Are barcode readers working properly? Again, it is critical to maintain the link between the imaging plate and patient information.
  - Inspect the laser printer for ink and paper. Make sure the printer is clean and the output bin is free of obstructions. If the printer can be used manually for copies, inspect the printer glass for dirt, fingerprints, and so on, and clean according to the manufacturer's specifications. Artifacts produced by dirt and fingerprints can appear and be interpreted as pathology, possibly resulting in false-positive diagnoses.

Box 12-1 *Daily QC Duties for Technologists*

Inspect and clean cassettes
Inspect hinge and latch
Erase imaging plates
Verify digital interfaces and network transmission
Inspect laser printer

Weekly (Box 12-2)

- Clean and inspect receptors
  - Clean CR cassettes as needed, and inspect DR image receptors for dirt or damage. Inspect the entire length of the DR cable for splits or exposure of wires. If breaks or wear has caused wire exposure, inform service personnel immediately. In addition to the danger of electrical shock to personnel, electrical shorts can cause failure of equipment and/or noise on the image.
- Equipment manufacturers should provide lists of appropriate system tests to be performed by the technologists. This type of testing may be performed by a designated QC technologist rather than by each individual technologist. Examples of this type of test are:
  - Image acquisition testing with phantoms
  - Cassette integrity testing with special, standardized cassettes
- Clean the air intakes on the CR reader.
  - Air is used to cool the reader electronics. If dirt and debris are allowed to clog the intakes, the reader could sustain serious damage. In addition, debris entering the air intake could obscure the lens of the scanning laser or reader mirrors and produce artifacts.
- Clean the cathode ray tube (CRT) screen, keyboard, and mouse.
  - With multiple people using digital imaging systems, and because the digital imaging system makes use of touch screen technology, CRT screens get dirty very quickly. Multiple users leave multiple fingerprints that, because of the oil in the skin, attract and retain dust and dirt particles. From a visual standpoint, it is much easier to view images on a screen not obscured by streaks and smears. From a health standpoint, many hands on the same surfaces without proper cleaning can lead to increased transmission of illness. Care must be taken to properly clean and disinfect these surfaces according to manufacturers' guidelines.
- All problems must be recorded and reported immediately.

Monthly (Box 12-3)

- Reject analysis
  - It is critical that repeat exposures are identified so that data concerning repeat reason, number of repeats, and the technologist responsible for the repeat can be analyzed. One issue is that whereas DR systems record the milliamperage seconds (mAs) and kilovoltage peak (kVp) values directly on the film, CR systems do not, nor do CR systems identify the technologist unless that information is input manually. In cases when the department does not require manual technologist identification input, it is strongly recommended that a personal

---

Box 12-2 *Weekly QC Duties for Technologists*

Clean and inspect receptors
Clean air intakes of CR reader
Clean CRT screen
Clean computer keyboard and mouse

Box 12-3 *Monthly QC Duties for Technologists*

Reject analysis
  Reject reasons
  Positioning errors
  Marker errors
  Equipment malfunction errors
Clean imaging plates
Artifact identification
Problem reporting

---

repeat rate log be kept by each technologist. Figure 12-1 is a sample log. Keeping a log helps the technologist see possible trends in exposure errors. For example, if the repeat reason is insufficient density (too light), the cause could be poor calibration of the automatic exposure control (AEC), or it could be poor imaging skills. Either way, identification of this trend allows the technologist to improve imaging procedures and better protect the patient. This can be accomplished to a certain extent with a software program. Many vendors have software to automatically keep repeats in a folder for the QC technologists to review, eliminating the issue of technologists deleting repeat exposure images.

■ QC out of standard images
  ● Typically, a technologist is assigned the responsibility of coordinating analysis of images of suboptimal quality. This may be done in concert with a radiation physicist, the purpose being to identify equipment and technologist performance errors. Figure 12-2 is a sample reject analysis form. This type of analysis helps determine:

Repeat Exam Log

Technologist: _____ Date: _____ Room # _____ Portable _____

Patient ID	Exam	Repeat Reason											
		Positioning	Overexposed	Underexposed	Reprinted	Motion	Wrong exam code	Over collimated	Artifact	No exposure	Double exposed	No marker	Marker over part	Other

Figure 12-1 Sample repeat examination log.

CR/DR Image Analysis Form

Exam/view _____ cm _____ kVp _____ mAs _____

Patient hx _____ Film _____ CR _____ DR _____

Room or reader _____ Date _____ Technologist _____

	Area to evaluate	Criteria	Pass	Reject
1.	**Image identification**			
		Institution name		
		Patient name or number		
		Date		
2.	**Radiographic markers and placement**			
		Present and accurate		
		Location and orientation		
		Superimposition		
3.	**Collimation and shielding**			
4.	**Patient artifacts**			
5.	**Imaging equipment, handling, or processing artifacts**			
6.	**Image sharpness, magnification, minification, and distortion**			
7.	**Positioning**			
	Film size and part/receptor alignment	Appropriate imaging plate size		
		Correct central ray placement		
	Angle	Tube/part angle is correct		
	Rotation	Part rotated correctly		
	Inclusion	All anatomy included		
8.	**Exposure**			
	kVp	Appropriate for type and amount of contrast		
	Scale of contrast	Black/white ratio appropriate		
	Density	Overall too dark/too light		
		Exposure index appropriate		
		mAs selection appropriate		
9.	**Equipment**	Reader error		
		Histogram error		
10.	**Accept/reject**			
Comments/action				

Figure 12-2 Sample image analysis/reject form.

- Reject reasons
    - This is fairly easy to identify in DR images because the mAs and kVp are recorded as part of the image. In CR, images that are out of the recommended exposure range can be identified, but unless the technical factors are manually input, there is no way to tell whether the problem was caused by mAs or kVp errors. Without the use of side/position markers, there is no way to positively link an image with the performing technologist.
    - Positioning errors should be easy to identify. Again, without input as to performing technologist, it will be difficult to identify skill issues. It is strongly recommended that the department put a procedure in place that accomplishes this, not for punitive purposes, but for standardization of exposure practices. A major part of being a professional in the imaging sciences is having the integrity to accept responsibility for one's own work. Positioning errors may also be the cause of incorrect processing, related to the position of the part on the imaging plate, collimation, or alignment resulting in poor images even if technique is correct. Vendors are developing software to minimize this, but software is no substitute for proper positioning, collimation, and alignment.
    - Side/position marker errors may be very difficult to identify. Because postexposure marking is easily done, technologists may not see the benefit of using personal identification (ID) markers. However, this may lead to serious errors that are difficult to identify. In one case, a technologist performed a portable chest x-ray on an infant. On processing, she noticed that her personal marker was on the wrong side of the chest. On investigation, she discovered that she had marked the chest correctly, but the infant had situs inversus that was never identified during six previous examinations because technologists had failed to use their personal ID markers. There is no substitute for using proper personal ID markers correctly. Incorrect or lack of use of side identification markers may result in legal complications if images are included in a court case. With no blocker for the technologist to use as an identifier of cassette and image orientation, there would be no way to prove proper marking without the technologist ID markers.
- Clean imaging plates
    - Image plates (IPs) should be removed from the cassette and inspected visually for dirt, hair, lint, scratches, or cracks. Weekly inspection is recommended, especially for departments with high throughput or frequent "dirty" case use. It is important that lint-free cotton gloves be worn to avoid further contaminating the IP. A lint-free cloth, such as a photographic lens cloth, should be used to gently wipe debris off the imaging plate surface. A camel hair brush can be used but should be stored so that dust and dirt do not collect on it. If this is ineffective, cleaning solutions can be used. Use only cleaning solutions specifically recommended by the manufacturer, and be sure to follow the material

safety data sheet (MSDS) guidelines provided by the cleaning solution distributor. If the artifact cannot be removed, the IP will have to be replaced.

- Imaging plate disposal
  - Imaging plates contain a small amount of barium, which must be discarded according to state and U.S. Environmental Protection Agency (EPA) regulations.
  - Disposal must be handled by a licensed disposal company; no other disposal, such as trashcans, is acceptable. This type of disposal requires an EPA identification number assigned by the state. Be familiar with disposal regulations.
    - Artifact identification
      - Monthly QC of images will help identify recurring artifacts caused by debris on IPs, cassettes, laser lenses, and reader mirrors. Major artifacts should be noted at the time of processing and reported. Smaller, less intrusive artifacts can be missed or ignored, resulting in long-term problems.
  - Proper problem reporting procedures provide a mechanism through which recurring quality trends can emerge. For example, if several reports are received from a particular room that images are excessively noisy or too light, the room may need to be inspected for system interference or AEC recalibration. It will also help service personnel determine what issues exist based on location and frequency.

Service Personnel Responsibilities (Box 12-4)

Although specific responsibilities vary from manufacturer to manufacturer and vendor to vendor, generally speaking, service personnel have a duty to the consumer to ensure that equipment is being maintained properly. This is accomplished through a program of **preventative maintenance (PM),** which typically takes place semiannually. Preventative maintenance consists of a series of equipment tests that are performed by a service engineer. This engineer may be employed by the hospital or the equipment manufacturer. Some of the PM duties are listed below:

- X-ray generator, tube, and reader
  - Tests are performed to establish accuracy and reproducibility. The code value at each pixel should accurately reflect the x-ray exposure at that location. Reproducibility of exposures produced should be ±2% within established exposure parameters measured in multiple exposures (Carestream [Rochester, NY] recommends 20 exposures per test at 80 kVp, filtration, nongrid, with three levels of exposure at the 0.1 mR, 1.0 mR, and 10 mR values).
  - If obvious low contrast dark or light bands are seen, then average densities are measured within these bands so that the recalibration can exclude them.
  - If high contrast white spots are seen, they usually indicate dust on the screen. If sharply defined white streaks are seen that are parallel to the slow scan direction and are identical in size, dust may have accumulated on the light-collection optics and will have to be cleaned by a service engineer.
- Phosphor accuracy testing

> **Box 12-4** *Service Personnel QC Responsibilities*
>
> **Preventative Maintenance**
> X-ray generator, tube
> CR reader
> Phosphor accuracy testing
> Image processing functions
> Image display testing
> Reader erasure functions
> Spatial frequency response testing

- This is accomplished by using a special standardized cassette that is not used for daily imaging procedures.
- Exposure is made to the imaging plate, and it is inspected for response uniformity and artifacts.
- Image processing
  - Image processing parameters are tested to ensure that anatomic image analysis and histogram production are operating correctly. Service personnel will disable all automatic functions and process an image manually. This results in particular code displays that allow the service personnel to look at each image parameter and evaluate it for processing errors. Test images should be discarded and not sent to archive storage space.
- Image display
  - Testing the system display verifies correct positioning and image processing selections. These images are subsampled so most detail is not present. These images are for image display issues only and should never be used for evaluating system performance.
- Screen erasure
  - To avoid interference from previous exposures that store light or signal, or from extraneous light sources in the reader, the erasure function of the reader must be tested at least once per year.
- Spatial frequency response testing
  - Line-pair testing phantoms are used to determine resolution patterns. These phantoms encase objects that are at least 0.05 mm in thickness and have patterns at least 10 mm in length. Manufacturers determine guidelines for maximum and minimum resolution standards.

Radiation Physicist Responsibilities (Box 12-5)

Schedules for physicist review of digital imaging systems may vary depending on availability. One physicist may handle multiple medical facilities, visiting each one on a weekly or monthly basis. Others may be employed by only one facility and be much more active in determining review procedures. Typical responsibilities include:

- Semiannual/annual

> **Box 12-5** *Radiation Physicist's Responsibilities*
>
> **Semiannual/Annual QC**
> Maintain base-line values
> Exposure trends
> Reject rate analysis
> QC record review
> Service history analysis

- Review of departmental images to:
  - Reestablish baseline values
  - Check exposure indicator's accuracy with calibrated ion chamber
  - Determine exposure trends
  - Analyze repeat rates
  - Review QC records
  - Analyze service history

The standard QC tests for filtration, collimation, focal-spot size, kVp calibration, exposure timer accuracy, exposure linearity, exposure reproducibility, and protective apparel will remain the same, but the American Association of Physicists in Medicine (AAPM) has established a set of QC parameters to be followed for photostimulable phosphor systems. AAPM Report 74 details the daily, weekly, monthly, semiannual, and annual tests and reports to be performed.

SUMMARY

- QC standards for image acquisition, processing, and equipment maintenance all contribute to TQM, or CQI.
- The radiologic technologist is the first line of defense in preventing, recognizing, and reporting QC issues.
- Radiologic technologists, service personnel, and radiation physicists each have a set of QC activities that they are responsible to maintain.

CHAPTER REVIEW QUESTIONS

1. How is total quality management used in digital imaging? Are there any new procedures or processes that did not exist with film/screen radiography?

2. What are the daily and weekly activities the imaging technologist needs to complete to ensure the highest quality imaging?

3. What monthly activities are the most important? Are there any that can be skipped? What would be the consequences of not completing these activities?

4. Why is it important to establish a repeat analysis database? What specific information could be gained from such a database?

5. Why are some activities designated specifically for the service engineer? What could be the result if someone other than the service engineer performed these activities?

6. What is at risk if proper problem reporting systems do not exist? How could a lack of knowledge about what to report and to whom impact you?

7. What are the major responsibilities of the radiation physicist?

8. What might happen if nobody is concerned about correctly making images?

9. How would knowing your personal repeat rate affect your work?

10. Why is it important to know how artifacts occur?

GLOSSARY

acceptance testing testing that occurs to ensure equipment or processes are functioning within acceptable limits

application service provider (ASP) company that provides outsourcing of archiving and management functions for a pay-per-use or pay-per-month charge

archive historical collection of images stored in PACS

archive query software function that allows historical information to be gathered from digital storage, such as multiple examinations, a range of dates, or by pathology

archive server consists of the physical storage device of the archive system; it commonly consists of two or three tiers of storage

artifacts avoidable extraneous information on the image that interferes or distracts from image quality

aspect ratio ratio of the width of the monitor to the height of the monitor

automatic data recognition processing mode in which the computer analyzes data according to set parameters

automatic rescaling occurs when exposure is greater or less than the optimal amount to produce a diagnostic image; it is the effort of the computer to "fix" exposure errors

backing layer soft polymer that protects the back of the cassette

barcode label label attached either to the cassette or to the imaging plate that identifies the plate for the purpose of matching the examination to the plate

barium fluorohalide photostimulable phosphor located in the imaging plate

basic input/output system (BIOS) contains a simple set of instructions for the computer to perform several basic functions, such as boot up, run hardware diagnostics, interpret keyboard signals, and so on

binary code machine language of 1s and 0s

bit single unit of data

burner device that burns data onto a CD or DVD

bus series of connections, controllers, and chips that creates the information highway of the computer

bus topology type of network setup in which each of the computers and network devices are connected to a single cable

byte made up of 8 bits and is the amount of memory needed to store one alphanumeric character

cassette rigid plastic housing for the imaging plate

central processing unit (CPU) small chip found on the motherboard that manipulates data sent from a program; brains of the computer

cesium iodide scintillator (CsI) newer type of amorphous silicon detector that uses a cesium iodide (CsI) scintillator; the scintillator is made by growing very thin crystalline needles (5 μm wide) that work as light-directing tubes, much like fiberoptics

charge-coupled device (CCD) coupling devices that act as cameras that link phosphor signals to a signal

client-based network similar to a server-based network, in that there is a centralized computer that controls the operations of the network, but rather than sending the entire original resource to the client for processing, the server processes the resource as requested by the client and returns only the results back to the client

client/server-based system PACS workflow where the images are sent directly to the archive server after acquisition and are centrally located

coaxial cable network communication medium that is similar to TV cable wiring

collimation type of wire that consists of a center wire surrounded by insulation and then a grounded shield of braided wire; the shield minimizes electrical and radio frequency interference

color layer area within the conductive layer where electrons are trapped

complementary metal oxide semiconductor (CMOS) special type of memory chip that uses a small rechargeable or lithium battery to retain information about the PC's hardware while the computer is turned off

computed radiography (CR) or cassette-based digital radiography is the digital acquisition modality that uses storage phosphor plates to produce projection images

computer programmable electronic device that can store, retrieve, and process data

conductive layer layer of material that will absorb and reduce static electricity

continuous quality improvement (CQI) alternative set of terms for total quality management that includes maintenance of equipment, image acquisition, and processing standards

contrast manipulation conversion of the digital image using contrast enhancement parameters

detective quantum efficiency (DQE) measurement of how efficiently a system converts x-ray input signal into a useful output image

detector size actual physical size, length and width, of the x-ray detector

DICOM digital imaging and communications in medicine; it is a global information technology standard that allows network communication between modality and PACS

digital imaging any imaging acquisition process that produces an electronic image that can be viewed and manipulated on a computer

digital radiography (DR) or cassette-less systems use an x-ray absorber material coupled to a flat panel detector or a charged-coupled device to form the image

digital versatile disk (DVD) digital storage device that can hold up to seven times more than the CD, which equates to about 9.4 (single-sided) to 17 GB (double-sided) of data; in a DVD, there are multiple layers of the polycarbonate plastic

direct capture digital radiography these devices convert the incident x-ray energy directly into an electrical signal, typically using a photoconductor as the x-ray absorber and a thin-film transistor as the signal collection area, and send the electrical signal to the computer for processing and viewing

direct conversion conversion of x-ray energy to electrical signals without the light-conversion step

disaster recovery complete copy of the archive housed in another location and immediately available if the front-line archive goes down for any reason

display workstation generally a display monitor where postprocessing occurs or where images can be viewed

distributed system PACS workflow where the acquisition modalities send the images to a designated reading station and possibly review stations

dot pitch measurement of how close the dots are located to one another within a pixel

dry imager printer that uses heat to develop the film

edge enhancement enhancement occurs when fewer pixels in the neighborhood are included in the signal average; the smaller the neighborhood, the greater the enhancement

error maintenance correction to equipment after errors have occurred

exposure index (EI) term used by Carestream to express exposure values

exposure indicator number numerical representation of the amount of exposure, usually the mean value

fiberoptic cable network communication medium that uses glass threads to transmit data on the network in the form of light

field effect transistor (FET) device within an imaging detector that isolates each pixel element and reacts like a switch to send the electrical charges to the image processor

file room workstation workstation found in the radiology file room that may be used to burn CDs or print films for outside use

film digitizer device that scans hard copy x-ray images and converts them to digital images

fixed mode postprocessing mode in which the user selects the exposure index: latitude is set by the menu selection; no histogram is generated, and there is no recognition of imaging plate division; the resultant image is a direct reflection of the exposure value

flat panel detector detector that consists of a photoconductor, which holds a charge on its surface that can then be read out by a thin-film transistor

focused grid grid in which the scatter absorbing lead lines are tilted so that at a prescribed distance, the lines will converge

grid frequency number of grid lines per inch

grid ratio ratio of the height of the grid line to the width of the interspace material

hanging protocol how a set of images will be displayed on the monitor

hard drive main repository for programs and documents on the computer

high-pass filtering technique for the enhancement of contrast and edge that amplifies the frequencies of areas of interest that are known (those frequencies that can be amplified) and suppresses frequencies outside the area of interest

histogram graphic representation of all of the digitally recorded signals of a digital x-ray exposure

HL-7 health level 7; standard protocol used for medical data systems

hospital information system (HIS) information system used throughout the hospital, includes direct patient care information, billing systems, and reporting systems

image annotation software function that allows text or markers to be digitally added to an image

image manager contains the master database of everything that is in the archive

image orientation identification of the top or side of an image

image sampling amount of information gathered from pixel storage

image stitching process of "sewing" together multiple images to form one continuous image

image storage process of sending the digital image to PACS or CD

imaging plate thin piece of plastic with several layers of material that capture and store image data

indirect capture digital radiography devices that absorb x-rays and convert them into light; the light is then detected by an area-charge-coupled device or thin-film transistor array in concert with photodiodes, and then converted into an electrical signal that is sent to the computer for processing and viewing

indirect conversion   two-step process in which x-ray photons are converted to light and then the light photons are converted to an electrical signal

kVp   kilovoltage peak

laser   amplification of stimulated emission of radiation, a device that creates and amplifies a narrow, intense beam of coherent light

latitude   amount of error that can be made in exposure factor choice and still result in the capture of a quality image

level   image manipulation parameter that changes screen image contrast usually through the use of a mouse

local area network (LAN)   small area networked with a series of cables or wireless access points so that the computers can share information and devices on the same network

logarithm of the median exposure (lgM)   term used by Agfa to express exposure to the imaging plate

look-up table (LUT)   reference histogram of the luminance values derived during image acquisition

low-pass filtering   result of averaging each pixel's frequency with surrounding pixel values to remove high frequency noise; the result is a reduction of noise and contrast; useful for viewing small structures such as fine bone

magnetic disk storage   short-term magnetic disk storage, usually found in arrays (RAID)

magneto-optical disk (MOD)   very similar to a CD or DVD in that it is read optically with a laser, but the disk itself is housed within a plastic cartridge

magnification   enlargement of an image in all dimensions without loss of sharpness

manual send   computer function that allows images to be sent to specified reading stations

mAs   milliamperage seconds

matrix   rectangular or square table of numbers that represent the pixel intensity to be displayed on the monitor

memory   used to store information being currently processed within the central processing unit

mesh topology   network that has multiple pathway interconnecting devices and networks

modulation transfer function   ability of a system to record available spatial frequencies

moiré   grid line or image noise pattern that occurs when either the alignment of the grid to the laser scan direction is incorrect or when spatial frequency is greater than the Nyquist frequency; a wraparound image will result

motherboard   largest circuitry board inside the computer; it contains many important small components to make the computer function properly

multiple manual selection mode   area of interest is selected by the technologist, and the image is derived from the selected areas imaged in semiautomatic mode

navigation functions   options available on the workstation that allow movement through menus, menu options, image processing choices, as well as movement through a series or stack of images and/or patient image folders

network   two or more objects sharing resources and information; interconnected computers, terminals, and servers connected by communication channels sharing data and program resources

network bridge   created so that larger networks can be segmented or broken up into smaller networks to reduce traffic within that network

network hub   central meeting point where cables from several devices can come together and share information throughout the group; it is a simple boxlike device with several wiring ports available to receive and pass on data to various pieces of equipment; the hub sends all information to every device connected.

network interface card (NIC)   interface between the computer and the network medium

network protocol   agreed-on set of rules for network communication

network router   device that can read portions of the messages and direct them to their intended target, even if the device is on a separate network and uses a different network protocol

network switch   similar to a hub but it sends data only to those devices to which the data are directed

Nyquist theorem   when sampling a signal such as the conversion from an analog to a digital image, the sampling frequency must be greater than twice the bandwidth of the input signal so that the reconstruction of the original image will be nearly perfect

operating system   software that controls the computer hardware and acts as a bridge between applications and the hardware

PACS   picture archival and communication system; consists of digital acquisition, display workstations, and storage devices interconnected through a network

PACS administrator   the person trained to oversee the PACS

patient demographics   input information regarding patient age, identifying number, ordering physician, and so on

peer-to-peer network   each computer on the network is considered equal; no computer has ultimate control over another

phosphor center   see *color layer*

phosphor layer   layer of photostimulable phosphor that "traps" electrons during exposure; usually made of phosphors from the barium fluorohalide family (e.g., barium fluorohalide, chlorohalide, or bromohalide crystals)

photometer device used to measure the luminescence of areas on the monitor

photomultiplier electronic device that amplifies light energy

photostimulable luminescence (PSL) light produced by a phosphor when struck by light or x-ray photons

photostimulable phosphor phosphor that produces light when stimulated by light or x-ray photons

picture archival and communication system networked group of computers, servers, and archives that can be used to manage digital images

pixel basic picture element on a display

port collection of connectors sticking out of the back of the computer that link adapter cards, drives, printers, scanners, keyboards and mice, and other peripherals that may be used

power supply delivers all electricity and provides connections to power devices in the computer

preventative maintenance (PM) periodic testing of equipment and materials before problem occurrence

protective layer very thin, tough, clear plastic covering in the imaging plate for protection of the phosphor layer

quality assurance another term for quality management, which is now considered antiquated; typically focuses on the person rather than the process

quality control (QC) subdivision of quality management that focuses on equipment functions

quality control (QC) station dedicated computer and monitor for the purpose of reviewing digital images

quantum mottle failure of an imaging system to record densities usually caused by a lack of x-ray photons

quantum noise recording error in the digital image

radiology information system (RIS) information system used in the radiology department for ordering examinations and reporting results

raster zigzag electron scanning pattern

reading station computer and monitor generally used by the physician interpreting the digital images

redundant array of independent disks (RAID) composed of several magnetic disks or hard drives that are linked together in an array

reflective layer layer in the imaging plate that sends light in a forward direction when released in the cassette reader; this may be black to reduce the spread of stimulating light and the escape of emitted light; some detail is lost in this process

refresh rate measure of how fast the monitor rewrites the screen or the number of times that the image is redrawn on the display each second

resolution number of pixels contained on a display

review workstation workstation used by other health care personnel to view radiology images

ring topology network in which the devices are connected in a circle

routine maintenance synonymous with preventive maintenance; maintenance of equipment that occurs before problem occurrences

S, sensitivity number term used by Fuji Medical to express exposure

semiautomatic mode postprocessing mode in which the latitude value of the histogram is fixed, and only a small reading area is used; there is no collimation detection, and the proper kV must be used to maintain subject contrast because the latitude value does not change

server computer that manages resources for other computers, servers, and networked devices

server-based network there is a centralized computer (server) that controls the operations, files, and sometimes the programs of the computers (clients) attached to the network

shuttering used to blacken out the white collimation borders in a digital image, effectively eliminating veil glare

smoothing also known as low-pass filtering, the result of averaging each pixel's frequency with surrounding pixel values to remove high frequency noise

softcopy reading images on the computer without hardcopy films

spatial frequency resolution amount of detail or sharpness in a digital image

speed in conventional radiography, *speed* is determined by the size and layers of crystals in the film and screen; computed radiography system "speeds" are a reflection of the amount of photostimulable luminescence given off by the imaging plate while being scanned by the laser

star topology network that has the devices connected to a central hub or switch

super user someone trained within the hospital to help troubleshoot and teach others to use the PACS

support layer semirigid material in the imaging plate that gives the imaging sheet some strength

system architecture hardware and software infrastructure of the system's workflow

tape magnetic tape cartridges used for long-term storage archives

teleradiology moving images via telephone lines to and from remote locations

The Joint Commission organization that accredits health care organizations, such as hospitals, clinics, and labs

thick-client computer that can work independently from the network and can process and manage its own files

thin-film transistor (TFT) photosensitive array, made up of small (about 100 to 200 μm) pixels, converts the light into electrical charges

thin-client device that is found on a network that requests services and resources from a server

tier level, layer, or division of something

topology physical (geometric) layout of the connected devices on a network

total quality management (TQM) see *continuous quality improvement*

twisted-pair wire network communication medium that consists of four twisted pairs of copper wire that are insulated and bundled together with an RJ-45 termination

ultra density optical disk (UDO) new generation MOD; uses blue laser technology in its read and write activities

viewable area measured from one corner of the display to the opposite corner diagonally

web-based system very similar to a client/server system with regard to how the data flow, but the biggest difference is that not only are the images held centrally but so is the application software for the client display

wet imager printer that uses chemicals to develop the film

wide area network (WAN) network that spans a large area, city, state, nation, continent, and/or world

window image manipulation parameter that changes screen image brightness usually through the use of a mouse

wircless network communication medium that uses either infrared or radio frequencies as its means of communication

workflow amount of work or examinations completed over a period of time

ABBREVIATION TABLE

µGy	microgray	**HIPAA**	Health Insurance Portability and Accountability Act
3D	three-dimensional	**HIS**	hospital information system
AAPM	American Association of Physicists in Medicine	**HL-7**	health level 7
AC	alternating current	**Hz**	hertz
ACR	American College of Radiology	**IDE**	integrated drive electronics
AEC	automatic exposure control	**IP**	internet protocol
AGP	accelerated graphics port	**IP**	image plate
AIT	advanced intelligent tape	**JPEG**	joint photographic expert group
a-Si:H	amorphous selenium	**keV**	kilo-electron-volt
ASP	application service provider	**kVp**	kilovoltage peak (prime)
BIOS	basic input/output system	**L**	latitude
C7-T1	refers to the junction of the seventh cervical vertebra and the first thoracic vertebra	**L5/S1**	refers to the junction of the fifth lumbar vertebra and the first section of the sacrum
CAD	computed aided diagnosis	**LAN**	local area network
cat 5	category 5	**LCD**	liquid crystal display
CCD	charge-coupled device	**lgM**	logarithm
CD	compact disk	**lp/mm**	line pairs per millimeter
cm	centimeter	**LTO**	linear tape open
CMOS	complementary metal oxide semiconductor	**LUT**	look-up table
CPU	central processing unit	**mAs**	milliamperage seconds
CQI	continuous quality management	**MB**	megabyte
CR	computed radiography	**MIP**	maximum intensity projection
CRT	cathode ray tube	**MOD**	magneto-optical disk
CT	computed tomography	**MPR**	multiplanar reconstruction
DAS	direct attached storage	**mR**	milliroentgen
DC	direct current	**MRI**	magnetic resonance imaging
DICOM	digital imaging and communications in medicine	**MSDS**	material data safety sheets
DLT	digital linear tape	**MTF**	modulation transfer function
DQE	detector quantum efficiency	**NAS**	network attached storage
DR	digital radiography	**NEMA**	National Electrical Manufacturers Association
DSA	digital subtraction angiography	**NIC**	network interface card
DVD	digital versatile disk	**nm**	nanometer
EI	exposure index	**OID**	object image distance
EMR	electronic medical record	**OS**	operating system
EPA	Environmental Protection Agency	**PACS**	picture archiving and communications system
eV	electron volt	**PC**	personal computer
FET	field effect transistor	**PCI**	peripheral component interconnect
GB	gigabyte	**PM**	preventative maintenance
GUI	graphical user interface	**PSL**	photostimulable luminescence

ABBREVIATION TABLE, CONT.

QA	quality assurance	**SQL**	structured query language
QC	quality control	**SSD**	shaded surface display
RAID	redundant array of independent disks	**TCP**	transmission control protocol
RAM	random access memory	**TFT**	thin-film transistor
RF	radio frequency	**TJC**	The Joint Commission
RIS	radiology information system	**TQM**	total quality management
S (number)	sensitivity	**UDO**	ultra density optical disk
SAN	storage area network	**UID**	unique identifiers
SCP	service class provider	**USB**	universal serial bus
SCSI	small computer system interface	**VRT**	volume rendering technique
SCU	service class user	**WAN**	wide area network
SOPs	service/object pairs		

Index

3D. *See* Three-dimensional reconstructions

A

AAPM. *See* American Association of Physicists in Medicine
AAPM Report No. 93, 214
Accelerated graphics ports (SGP), 25
Acceptance testing, 197
Acquisition errors, 106
Active layer, 64, 67*f. See also* Phosphor layer
ADC. *See* Analog-to-digital converters
Adhesive tape, artifacts and, 90, 90*f*
Administrator, 210
Advanced intelligent tape (AIT), 176
Advanced Micro Devices (AMD), 24
AEC. *See* Automatic exposure controls
Agfa systems, 86, 87*f*
AGP. *See* Accelerated graphics ports
Air intakes, 216, 216*b*
AIT. *See* Advanced intelligent tape
Aliasing, 111, 113*f. See also* Moiré pattern
AMD. *See* Advanced Micro Devices
American Association of Physicists in Medicine (AAPM), 198-205, 200*f*, 214, 222
American College of Radiology, 55, 214
American National Standards Institute (ANSI), 58
Amorphous silicon detectors, 9*f*, 101
Analog, defined, 72
Analog-to-digital converters (ADC), 5, 73
Angle measurement, 156
Annotation, 121, 123*f*, 154, 155*f*
ANSI. *See* American National Standards Institute
Antistatic material, 64, 66*f*
Application service providers (ASP), 178-180, 180*f*
Architecture, 139-142, 140*f*, 141*f*, 142*f*
Archive query function, 125. *See also* Queries
Archive servers
    long-term storage and, 171-173, 173*f*
    magnetic disks and, 176-178, 178*f*
    optical disks and, 173-175, 174*f*, 175*f*
    overview of, 135, 136*f*, 168
    short-term storage and, 169-171, 169*f*, 170*f*, 171*f*, 172*f*, 173*f*
    tape and, 175-176, 176*f*, 177*f*
Archives
    considerations for, 178-180, 179*f*, 180*f*
    image manager and, 167-168, 168*f*
    overview of, 166-167, 166*f*, 167*f*
Artifacts
    aliasing and, 111, 113*f*
    grid selection and, 83, 84*f*
    imaging plates and, 88-90, 89*f*, 90*f*, 91*f*

Artifacts *(Continued)*
    operator error and, 94-95, 94*f*, 95*f*
    overview of, 88
    plate readers and, 90-93, 91*f*, 92*f*, 93*f*
    printers and, 94
    quality control and, 215, 215*b*, 217*b*, 220
    quantum mottle as, 82, 82*f*, 94, 113, 114
a-silicon. *See* Amorphous silicon detectors
ASP. *See* Application service providers
Aspect ratios, defined, 34
Automatic data recognition, 87
Automatic exposure controls (AEC), 82, 217
Automatic rescaling, 113

B

Background removal, 120, 120*f*
Backing layer, 66, 67*f*
Backscatter, 90, 91*f*
Backups, 189
Barcode labels, 67, 68*f*, 215, 215*b*
Barium fluorohalide, 10-11, 12, 64, 220
Basic input/output systems. *See* BIOS
Batteries, 28
Binary code, 20, 21*f*, 22*f*
BIOS (basic input/output systems), 25
Bit depth, 73
Bits, 20
Boxes, 21, 23*f*
Bridges, 51
Brightness, 73, 119
Bucky apparatus, 4, 83
Burning, 32, 158, 189-191, 190*f*
Bus mice, 32
Bus networks, 53, 53*f*
Buses, 25
Bytes, 20

C

Cables, 48-49, 48*f*, 49*f*
CAD. *See* Computer aided diagnosis
Capp, M. Paul, 8
Carestream, 86, 87*f*, 114, 115*f*
Cassette-based digital radiography. *See* Computed radiography (CR)
Cassettes
    overview of, 64, 65*f*, 66*f*
    quality control and, 215, 215*b*, 216
Cathode ray tube (CRT) monitors
    overview of, 33, 34, 35*f*, 37*t*, 143, 145*f*
    quality control and, 202, 216*b*
CCD (charge coupled devices), 7-8, 9*f*, 102, 103*f*
CCD film digitizers, 186, 186*f*
CD (compact disks), 31-32, 31*f*, 151, 158, 189-191, 190*f*
CD/DVD drives, 31-32, 31*f*

Central processing units. *See* CPU
Cesium iodide (CsI) scintillators, 102, 102*f*, 103*f*
Charged coupled devices. *See* CCD
Chemical laser imagers, 187*f*, 188, 205-206
Cine function, 153
Client-based networks, 46-47, 46*f*
Clients, computers as, 47
Client/server-based systems, 139-140, 140*f*
Close patient (study) icon, 153-154
CMOS (complementary metal oxide semiconductors), 28, 104
Coaxial cables, 48, 48*f*
Collimation
    artifacts and, 94, 94*f*, 95*f*
    overview of, 84-85, 85*f*
    quality control and, 222
    shuttering and, 120, 120*f*
Color layer, 66, 67*f*
Communication, networks and, 52
Complementary metal oxide semiconductors. *See* CMOS
Component role network classification, 43-47, 45*f*, 46*f*
Compression, 58
Compression recall, 208-209
Compton interactions (scatter), 84, 94*f*
Computed radiography (CR)
    cassettes and, 64, 65*f*, 66*f*
    image sampling and, 110-111, 112*f*
    imaging plates and, 64-68, 67*f*
    overview of, 5, 6-7, 6*f*, 7*f*
    readers and, 68-75, 70*f*, 71*f*, 72*f*, 110
Computed tomography (CT) scans, 4, 5*f*
Computer aided diagnosis (CAD), 187
Computers
    BIOS and, 25
    boxes and, 21, 23*f*
    bus and, 25
    CD/DVD drives and, 31-32, 31*f*
    CMOS and, 28
    CPU and, 24, 24*f*, 25*f*
    hard drive and, 30-31, 31*f*
    memory and, 26, 26*f*
    monitors and, 33-36, 35*f*, 37*t*
    motherboard and, 21, 23*f*
    network cards and, 28, 29*f*
    networks and, 47, 47*f*
    operating systems and, 36-38
    overview of, 20, 20*f*, 21*f*, 22*f*
    peripherals and, 32-33
    ports and, 27-28, 27*f*
    power supply and, 28-30, 30*f*
    radiology department and, 38
    sound cards and, 28
Conductive layer, 65, 67*f*

Page references followed by "*f*" indicate figures, by "*t*" indicate tables, and by "*b*" indicate boxes.

233